Home-Based Medical Care for Older Adults

Jessica L. Colburn
Bruce Leff
Jennifer Hayashi
Mattan Schuchman

Editors

Home-Based Medical Care for Older Adults

A Clinical Case Book

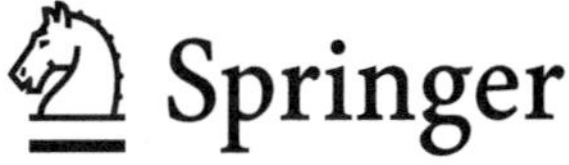
Springer

Editors
Jessica L. Colburn
Division of Geriatric Medicine
and Gerontology
Johns Hopkins University
Baltimore, MD
USA

Jennifer Hayashi
Smyth Building
MedStar House Call Program
Baltimore, MD
USA

Bruce Leff
Division of Geriatric Medicine
Johns Hopkins University
Baltimore, MD
USA

Mattan Schuchman
Johns Hopkins University
Baltimore, MD
USA

ISBN 978-3-030-23482-9   ISBN 978-3-030-23483-6   (eBook)
https://doi.org/10.1007/978-3-030-23483-6

This Springer imprint is published by the registered company Springer Nature Switzerland AG
The registered company address is: Gewerbestrasse 11, 6330 Cham, Switzerland

To our patients and their caregivers, who are our best teachers,

and

To our greatest mentors, Dr. John R. Burton and Dr. William B. Greenough, III, who taught us how to listen to our patients and their caregivers.

Foreword

Geriatric Home-Based Medical Care

In healthcare practice of the twentieth century, we have placed the high technology modern hospital as the best way to treat most serious illnesses. For older individuals, however, the hospital has many substantial hazards, such as delirium, falls, antibiotic-resistant infections, and superinfections created by antibiotics such as *C. difficile*.

There is little evidence that lives are saved by hospitalization for many conditions that can be more safely and effectively treated at home. Examples of these are pneumonia and less serious lower respiratory infections, congestive heart failure, skin infections, cellulitis, volume depletion (diarrhea, heat sweat losses), as well as the overexuberant use of diuretics and salt-wasting renal conditions.

We know and have clearly demonstrated that patients and their families prefer medical care at home and are usually capable of learning and carrying out nursing tasks and often higher technology tasks. How to provide home-based primary care is nicely outlined in this book. However, finding a way to transmute the funds currently devoted to hospital-centered care into home-based primary care will challenge hospitals and health systems alike.

To accomplish this goal will require a major shift which, when realized, will result in much improved healthcare for older people. With advanced technologies now available, we will be able to deliver the most effective treatments and diagnostics to the patient at home and not force frail older patients to make the hazardous journey to the hospital.

William B. Greenough III, MD, FACP
Division of Geriatric Medicine & Gerontology
Johns Hopkins School of Medicine
Baltimore, MD, USA

Preface

This book uses a patient-focused, case-based approach to address the common challenges faced by home-based medical care physicians and teams caring for homebound older adults. Home-based medical care is growing in scope, and there is now an expanding evidence base, due to the increase in home-based medical programs, the Independence at Home Demonstration projects, and the growing research focused on an array of home-based care delivery models. As the demand for home-based medical care continues to grow, there is a need for providers to be able to address the unique needs of patients receiving care at home. Our recent textbook focused on home-based medical care was well received, and we received feedback that a specific, case-based approach would be of value for home-based providers. This book aims to assist those providers with evidence-based approaches to common problems.

Baltimore, MD, USA Jessica L. Colburn, MD
Jennifer Hayashi, MD
Bruce Leff, MD
Mattan Schuchman, MD

Contents

Contributors

Karen Abrashkin, MD Northwell Health House Calls Program, New Hyde Park, NY, USA

Elizabeth Arrabito, MSN, RN-BC, FNP-BC Departments of Medical Utilization and Care Management, Healthfirst, Inc., New York, NY, USA

Shahla Baharlou, MD Icahn School of Medicine at Mount Sinai, New York, NY, USA

Sonica Bhatia, MD The Mount Sinai Health System, New York, NY, USA

Jessica L. Colburn, MD Johns Hopkins University School of Medicine, Division of Geriatric Medicine & Gerontology, Baltimore, MD, USA

Thomas K. M. Cudjoe, MD, MPH Johns Hopkins University School of Medicine, Division of Geriatric Medicine & Gerontology, Baltimore, MD, USA

Konstantinos Deligiannidis, MD, MPH, FAAFP Northwell Health House Calls Program, New Hyde Park, NY, USA

Christian Escobar, MD Department of Medicine, Department of Geriatrics and Palliative Medicine, Icahn School of Medicine at Mount Sinai, New York, NY, USA

Thomas E. Finucane, MD Johns Hopkins University School of Medicine, Division of Geriatric Medicine & Gerontology, Baltimore, MD, USA

Joseph Graziano, MS, PT Johns Hopkins Home Care Group, Baltimore, MD, USA

Jennifer Hayashi, MD MedStar House Call Program, Baltimore, MD, USA

Cameron R. Hernandez, MD Department of Medicine, Department of Geriatrics and Palliative Medicine, Icahn School of Medicine at Mount Sinai, New York, NY, USA

Abigail Holley Houts, MD Minnesota Department of Human Services, St. Paul, MN, USA

Namirah Jamshed, MD UT Southwestern Medical Center, Dallas, TX, USA

Fay Kahan, LCSW Mount Sinai Health System, New York, NY, USA

Rachel Kaplan, RN Northwell Health House Calls Program, New Hyde Park, NY, USA

Bruce Kinosian, MD Division of Geriatric Medicine, Perelman School of Medicine, University of Pennsylvania, Philadelphia, PA, USA

Fred C. Ko, MD Departments of Geriatrics and Palliative Medicine and Medicine, Icahn School of Medicine at Mount Sinai, New York, NY, USA

M. Victoria M. Kopke, MD The Mount Sinai Health System, New York, NY, USA

Sarah Koppel, LCSW Mount Sinai Medical System, New York, NY, USA

Bruce Leff, MD Johns Hopkins University School of Medicine, Division of Geriatric Medicine & Gerontology, Baltimore, MD, USA

Sharon A. Levine, MD Massachusetts General Hospital, Boston, MA, USA

Ina Li, MD Clinical Director, Continuum of Care and Home Based Services, Christiana Care Health System, Wilmington, DE, USA

Elizabeth McCormick, MD Mount Sinai Visiting Doctors Program, Departments of Medicine & Geriatrics and Palliative Medicine, Icahn School of Medicine at Mount Sinai, New York, NY, USA

Yasmin S. Meah, MD, CWSP Departments of Medicine, Medical Education, Geriatrics and Palliative Medicine, Icahn School of Medicine at Mount Sinai, New York, NY, USA

Melissa Morgan-Gouveia, MD Department of Medicine, Christiana Care Health System, Newark, DE, USA

Division of Geriatrics and Gerontology, Johns Hopkins University School of Medicine, Baltimore, MD, USA

Linsey O'Donnell, DO Clinical Lead, Community-based Supportive and Palliative Care Program, Christiana Care Health System, Wilmington, DE, USA

Jonathan Ripp, MD, MPH Icahn School of Medicine at Mount Sinai, New York, NY, USA

Monika Robinson, DrOT, OTR/L Department of Occupational Therapy, Midwestern University, Downers Grove, IL, USA

Mattan Schuchman, MD Johns Hopkins University School of Medicine, Baltimore, MD, USA

Cindy Seidenman, PT, DPT John Hopkins Home Care Group, Lutherville, MD, USA

Sarah L. Szanton, PhD, ANP, FAAN John Hopkins School of Nursing, Baltimore, MD, USA

Ania Wajnberg, MD Icahn School of Medicine at Mount Sinai, New York, NY, USA

Katherine Wang, MD Icahn School of Medicine at Mount Sinai, New York, NY, USA

Mia Yang, MD Wake Forest School of Medicine, Winston Salem, NC, USA

Megan E. Young, MD Boston University School of Medicine, Boston, MA, USA

Jean Yudin, MSN, GNP Schnable In Home Primary Care Program, Division of Geriatric Medicine, Perelman School of Medicine, University of Pennsylvania, Philadelphia, PA, USA

Erin Zahradnik, MD University of Chicago, Chicago, IL, USA

Meng Zhang, MD Mount Sinai Visiting Doctors Program, Departments of Medicine & Geriatrics and Palliative Medicine, Icahn School of Medicine at Mount Sinai, New York, NY, USA

Rachel Zimmer, DNP Wake Forest School of Medicine, Winston Salem, NC, USA

Chapter 1
Involuntary Weight Loss

Bruce Leff

Case Study

You recently joined a home-based medical care practice and assumed the care of Ms. F, an 84-year-old woman who is homebound because of severe osteoarthritis of her knees and hips.

Prior to your initial visit, you review her record. Her past medical history is notable for chronic heart failure, hypertension, hyperlipidemia, 10-pack-year cigarette use (discontinued 50 years prior), and gout.

She is a former secretary with a high-school education. She lives alone in an apartment. Her daughter who lives nearby visits two to three times a week and brings microwaveable food for her to heat up. Her daughter called you the day before the visit to give you an update on her status. She is concerned that Ms. F has been losing weight and not

B. Leff (✉)
Johns Hopkins University School of Medicine, Division of Geriatric Medicine & Gerontology, Baltimore, MD, USA
e-mail: bleff@jhmi.edu

J. L. Colburn et al. (eds.), *Home-Based Medical Care for Older Adults*, https://doi.org/10.1007/978-3-030-23483-6_1

eating as well over the past 4–6 months. In addition, she is concerned that over the past 12–18 months, her mother's memory is declining. Her short-term memory is deteriorating, and she seems to be having trouble managing her finances. She has also found some of the meals she has prepared for her mother in the trash, uneaten. Sometimes when she calls Ms. F on the phone, it takes her a few seconds to figure out that it is her daughter on the phone. She feels that her mother's mood is fine.

When you see the patient in her home, she has no specific complaints except that she says her daughter says she is losing weight and notes that her appetite is OK. She denies oral issues, dysphagia, abdominal pain, diarrhea, cardiopulmonary symptoms, or systemic symptoms. She is sleeping well, enjoys watching TV, and reports that her mood is "OK."

Her medications are atorvastatin, losartan, furosemide, aspirin, and acetaminophen. There have been no recent changes or additions.

Physical Examination

Thin older woman in pajamas and robe and in no distress.

VS: BP 143/87 mm Hg, HR 92 beats per minute, RR 16, and afebrile. Weight is 125 lbs., down from 132 lbs. at visit 3 months ago and 138 lbs. at visit 6 months ago. Head and neck examination is normal, with well-fitting dentures and no lymphadenopathy. She needs to push off substantially on the arms of her chair to get to standing position. She walks slowly, but steadily, with good balance. Apart from significant osteoarthritic changes in her knees, the remainder of the physical examination including neurological and breast exam is normal. She declined a rectal examination. She is awake, alert, and attentive. She has some word-finding trouble and occasionally repetitive speech.

Mini-Mental State Examination – 21/30.

Inspection of her home is notable for being mildly unkempt. There are dirty dishes in the sink and not much food in the refrigerator. Several frozen meals are in the freezer. There is no alcohol in the home. When you ask the patient to demonstrate how she uses the microwave to prepare her meals, she demurs.

When you ask Ms. F about addressing her weight loss, she tells you to discuss it with her daughter.

My Management

You obtain blood samples for a complete blood count, comprehensive metabolic panel, and thyroid stimulating hormone level, which were all within normal limits. She had a chest X-ray 6 months ago during a hospitalization for congestive heart failure, which was normal except for findings consistent with that acute exacerbation of her congestive heart failure.

Which of the following is the next best step to recommend to the patient's daughter?

A. Colonoscopy.
B. Mammogram.
C. Abdominal ultrasound.
D. Abdominal/pelvic CT scan.
E. Esophagogastroduodenoscopy (EGD).
F. Home health aide or friend for feeding; monitor clinically, and repeat history and physical examination within 6 months.
G. Prescribe appetite stimulant.

Diagnosis and Assessment

Involuntary weight loss (IWL) is a common problem among older adults. In community-based studies, approximately 1/3 of older adults lost at least 4% of their body weight over the course of a year [1]. There have been relatively few studies of the etiology of IWL, and most of these have been hospital-based, in referred populations. In these studies, people referred with IWL are put through an exhaustive workup to determine the etiology of the weight loss. These studies have been relatively consistent: approximately 1/4 of patients will have a psychiatric cause identified (usually depression or anxiety), and approximately 1/2 will have a physical cause identified, with malignancy and benign gastrointestinal causes as the most common. After an exhaustive workup, approximately 1/4 won't have a cause identified [2–4].The data suggest that in the absence of a specific complaint to guide a workup, an abdominal ultrasound or abdominal pelvic CT scan may be reasonable [5], but blind testing is otherwise not appropriate. Several studies suggest that when the patient has no specific complaints, a negative physical examination, and negative initial laboratory examination and chest radiograph, watchful waiting and serial evaluation are reasonable [6, 7].

Medications are a common cause in older adults [8]. There have been no studies of the etiology of IWL among home-bound older adults. However, in this population it is critical to consider social factors as potential contributors to IWL. Such factors include access to food, social isolation, and development of frailty syndrome. In addition, Alzheimer's dementia is also a cause of IWL. Weight loss commonly precedes clinical recognition of the dementia and may be related to deficits in executive function or to the underlying dementia itself [9, 10]. Finally, in patients with multiple chronic conditions and functional impairments, the etiology of IWL can be multifactorial.

Management

You call Ms. F's daughter and confirm the patient's weight loss. In addition, you tell her that you believe her mother has probable Alzheimer's disease; she says she suspected this. She asks you what is causing the weight loss and what should be done about it. You tell her that you think her mother's IWL is most likely due to her dementia and associated deficits in executive function that may be contributing to decreased food intake and weight loss. You recommend that provisions be made to help the patient with feeding – a friend or home health aide or that she or another family member help the patient more with eating, if possible. Further you tell her that you will remain vigilant and monitor her for new complaints to target a workup for a physical cause of weight loss and monitor her physical exam and basic labs. She is agreeable to this plan but says based on your explanation of the literature noted above, she would like her mother to have an abdominal imaging study. She asked whether an appetite stimulant would be useful for her mother. You tell her that while appetite stimulants, e.g., megestrol acetate, may result in several pounds of weight gain, that they are not associated with a mortality benefit and have substantial potential negative side effects and that you would not recommend their use in this situation.

Outcome

Ms. F's family devoted more time to helping the patient with meals and also hired a friend to do so. Over the next year, the patient continued to lose weight, though at a slower rate than previously. Ms. F's daughter remained concerned about another possible underlying cause of IWL; an abdominal ultrasound was obtained at a local imaging center and was negative. Her dementia steadily worsened. She died 3 years later with serial examinations over that time revealing no other causes of IWL.

Clinical Pearls and Pitfalls

- IWL is common in community-dwelling older adults, especially those with multiple chronic conditions and frailty.

- IWL is associated with dementia and may precede the diagnosis of dementia.
- Social and functional issues can contribute to IWL; assessment of a patient's home situation can help to identify contributing causes and approaches to treat or ameliorate IWL.
- In studies of the causes of IWL (mostly in referred population and most not among frail older adults), approximately 1/4 of patients will have a psychiatric cause identified (usually depression), 1/4 won't have a cause identified after an exhaustive workup, and approximately 1/2 will have a physical cause identified. Malignancy and benign gastrointestinal causes are the most common. Medications are a common cause in older adults. Watchful waiting and clinical surveillance in the absence of specific symptoms and negative initial workup are appropriate.
- Appetite stimulants should not be prescribed in the setting of IWL.

References

1. Ritchie CS, Joshipura K, Silliman RA, et al. Oral health problems and significant weight loss among community-dwelling older adults. J Gerontol A Biol Sci Med Sci. 2000;55(7):M366–71.
2. Rabinovitz M, Pitlik SD, Leifer M, et al. Unintentional weight loss. A retrospective analysis of 154 cases. Arch Intern Med. 1986;146(1):186–7.
3. Lankisch P, Gerzmann M, Gerzmann JF, Lehnick D. Unintentional weight loss: diagnosis and prognosis. The first prospective follow-up study from a secondary referral centre. J Intern Med. 2001;249(1):41–6.
4. Marton KI, Sox HC Jr, Krupp JR. Involuntary weight loss: diagnostic and prognostic significance. Ann Intern Med. 1981;95(5):568–74.
5. Hernández JL, Riancho JA, Matorras P, González-Macías J. Clinical evaluation for cancer in patients with involuntary weight loss without specific symptoms. Am J Med. 2003;114(8):631–7.

6. Metalidis C, Knockaert DC, Bobbaers H, Vanderschueren S. Involuntary weight loss. Does a negative baseline evaluation provide adequate reassurance? Eur J Intern Med. 2008;19(5):345–9.
7. Moriguti JC, Moriguti EK, Ferriolli E, et al. Involuntary weight loss in elderly individuals: assessment and treatment. Sao Paulo Med J. 2001;119(2):72–7.
8. Thompson MP, Morris LK. Unexplained weight loss in the ambulatory elderly. J Am Geriatr Soc. 1991;39(5):497–500.
9. Stewart R, Masaki K, Xue QL, et al. A 32-year prospective study of change in body weight and incident dementia: the Honolulu-Asia Aging Study. Arch Neurol. 2005;62(1):55–60.
10. White H, Pieper C, Schmader K. The association of weight change in Alzheimer's disease with severity of disease and mortality: a longitudinal analysis. J Am Geriatr Soc. 1998;46(10):1223–7.

Chapter 2
Assessing Decision-Making Capacity

Sharon A. Levine and Megan E. Young

Case Study

You are called by the building manager of a senior housing building. The building manager explains that your patient Ms. R has been cooking using a hot plate and has left the hot plate on all night. The home health aide (HHA) found it on this morning with an oven mitt on top with scorch marks and a hole burned into it. The stove in the apartment was disconnected by the building manager last month because Ms. R had set a small fire on the stove and burned the pot.

Ms. R is a 91-year-old woman who has been living in her own apartment in this building for 5 years. She has diabetes, hypertension, mild dementia, and peripheral vascular disease. Medications include aspirin, acetaminophen, glargine insulin, and vitamin D. She is allergic to lisinopril. Her daughter cares

S. A. Levine (✉)
Massachusetts General Hospital, Boston, MA, USA
e-mail: Slevine9@mgh.harvard.edu

M. E. Young
Boston University School of Medicine, Boston, MA, USA

© Springer Nature Switzerland AG 2020
J. L. Colburn et al. (eds.), *Home-Based Medical Care for Older Adults*, https://doi.org/10.1007/978-3-030-23483-6_2

for her own ill husband but does the grocery shopping and is Ms. R's health-care proxy. The patient has two grandchildren who are not involved and one son who lives 30 minutes away. She has a daily personal care/homemaker who comes for 4 hours in the morning. The HHA leaves at noon, and Ms. R is alone for the remainder of the day. Ms. R has expressed a strong desire to continue to cook and to live independently in her apartment. Although she has memory impairment, she has been able to make decisions about food preference and what clothing she wants to wear.

My Management

Which of the following is the next best step in Ms. R's management?

A. Admit her to a nursing home for safety.
B. Assess her decision-making capacity.
C. Remove the hot plate.
D. Pursue legal guardianship.

Diagnosis and Assessment

The first step is to assess decision-making capacity. To assess capacity, Ms. R has to be able to state the nature of the problem with keeping her hot plate, to discuss the risks and benefits, and to apply them to the specific decision regarding safety [1]. In this case you would ask the patient: "What are the dangers of having a hot plate in the house if your memory is not as good as it used to be?" Answers such as "I could forget to turn it off and burn something"; "I could start a fire and other residents of the building could get hurt"; or "I could burn something on the stove" demonstrate that she knows the risks. The next step is to see if she can apply the risks to the specific decision to remove her hot plate and if she can determine alternatives. You should ask, "Knowing that those risks are a possibility, what are the alternatives to the hot plate?", and review her alternative solutions. Answers to questions such as "What will you do if we take away the hot plate?" will indicate if she appreciates the situation. If she can answer these questions with well-reasoned answers such as "without a hot plate I would need someone to cook for me," the next step would be to ask "will you allow us to remove the hot plate?" If she answers "No, because I will not burn anything," she demonstrates her inability to apply risks to the situation. If she answers "Yes, if you can get someone to cook my meals," she demonstrates that she can appreciate the risks and apply them to her situation [1].

Management

Assessing her decision-making capacity will demonstrate if Ms. R can manipulate information, reason coherently, and appreciate the risks and benefits of continuing to use the hot plate, including potential dire consequences of harming her neighbors. Removing the hot plate and putting a homemaker in place who could cook preferred foods would provide a solution that preserves her autonomy and respects her choice to continue to live alone – with the exception of removing her ability to cook. This approach would demonstrate beneficence toward her without creating potential harm or maleficence to her or others.

Moving the patient to a nursing home – a much more restrictive environment – is not necessary at this stage. If the patient/family had resources and the patient agreed to leave her home, an assisted living community might be a good solution because of congregate meals. However, it would not preserve her autonomy for her preference to stay at home. Removing the hot plate without putting in place a homemaker would require home-delivered meals but is probably more restrictive than having someone cook food that meets Ms. R's preferences.

In this case, the high risk of harm to others requires a higher standard of certainty with respect to her decision-making capacity. If the patient does not meet this threshold, it may be time to consider legal intervention such as obtaining power of attorney or legal guardianship. A full assessment of medical and financial decision-making would be necessary to invoke power of attorney or legal guardianship, both of which are legal actions [2].

Outcome

In Ms. R's case, she is not able to state what the risks are to her and to others. When asked about the dangers of having a hot plate, she responds, "I didn't leave the hot plate on." When you show her the burnt oven mitt, she states, "I would never burn anything." Repeat Mini-Mental State Exam revealed a score of 20/30, which is 5 points lower than 2 years prior. You contact the patient's daughter to inform her that although Ms. R has the capacity to make decisions about what kinds of food she would like to eat and when she wants to eat, her cognitive functioning is getting worse, and she no longer has the capacity to use a stove or hot plate because she cannot state the risks and benefits in her situation. Furthermore, she is putting others at risk because she lives in a senior building. Her daughter agrees with you and states she has been worried about the hot plate as well. You agree to remove the hot plate from the apartment. You work with a nurse case manager in your practice to divide up the patient's personal care/home-maker hours so that someone can come for a shorter time in the morning to help with patient care and to prepare breakfast and lunch and then return in the late afternoon to make dinner. You arrange for home-delivered meals on the weekends.

Clinical Pearls and Pitfalls

- Capacity is decision-specific and it is a continuum. For a high-risk decision, there is a higher standard for certainty of capacity; for a low-risk decision, there is a lower standard.
- There are legal implications of causing harm to others (driving, fire, housing rules).
- It is important to provide as much independence in the least restrictive environment.
- It is helpful to link decision-making capacity to ethical concepts (autonomy, non-maleficence, justice, beneficence). For instance, autonomy is linked to living in the least restrictive environment as is pointed out in the case.

References

1. Tunzi M. Can the patient decide? Evaluating patient capacity in practice. Am Fam Physician. 2001;64:299–306.
2. Moye J, Marston C. Assessment of decision-making capacity in older adults: an emerging area of practice and research. J Gerontol B Psychol Sci Soc Sci. 2007;62:P3–P11.

Chapter 3
Acute Illness at Home

Abigail Holley Houts

Case Study

Mr. S is a 78-year-old man whom you follow in your home-based primary care practice. He calls your office to report a several-week history of worsening dyspnea on exertion. He was previously ambulatory (though with difficulty) within his apartment using a four-pronged cane but today became short of breath just walking the few steps from his bedroom to his bathroom. He has a history of stroke with resultant left hemiparesis and mild cognitive impairment, coronary artery disease with profoundly abnormal adenosine sestamibi stress test being treated pharmacologically, non-systolic congestive heart failure, gout, chronic hepatitis C, and Stage 3 chronic kidney disease. Medications include aspirin, carvedilol, furosemide, atorvastatin, albuterol, and allopurinol. He lives with his cousin and his cousin's three young grandchildren in a second-floor walk-up apartment. For just the last 2 weeks, a nurse has been setting up his medications in a pillbox for him. He is

A. H. Houts (✉)
Minnesota Department of Human Services, St. Paul, MN, USA
e-mail: Abigail.H.Houts@state.mn.us

© Springer Nature Switzerland AG 2020

J. L. Colburn et al. (eds.), *Home-Based Medical Care for Older Adults*, https://doi.org/10.1007/978-3-030-23483-6_3

independent in ADLs, although with difficulty. He has a history of alcohol and tobacco abuse, with a 40-pack-year smoking history. He quit both at the time of his stroke 7 years ago. In addition to dyspnea on exertion today, he does endorse some shortness of breath at rest and when attempting to lie flat at night. He denies chest pain, pressure, or discomfort. He reports that his chronic lower extremity edema has not worsened recently. He does feel that he has been gaining weight, however, particularly in his abdomen. He has not been febrile and denies coughing or wheezing. There are no changes to his bowel or urinary pattern. He has a Physician Order for Life-Sustaining Treatment (POLST) form that indicates his wishes are to be resuscitated and/or intubated for any acute, potentially reversible illnesses but also notes that his strong preference is to remain at home and avoid hospitalization if symptoms can be adequately controlled. He does not wish to go to the emergency department (ED) at this time but feels he will have no choice if you cannot help him.

My Management

What is your first step in the care of the patient?

A. Ask to speak with patient's cousin and advise him to call 911 immediately.
B. Tell patient you can order a chest X-ray and some blood tests to be done at home today.
C. Advise patient to double his furosemide dose and plan to call him tomorrow for an update.
D. Call patient's home health nurse and ask her to call you with a clinical assessment after her visit next week.

Diagnosis and Assessment

The correct answer is B. Mr. S's symptoms and past medical history create a large differential diagnosis for multiple potentially life-threatening etiologies. Additionally, his history of stroke with resultant cognitive impairment may make obtaining an accurate history challenging. He has only had nursing assistance in setting up his medications for the past 2 weeks, so medication adherence may be called into question. While his orthopnea may point toward a CHF exacerbation, he has not noted a significant change in his chronic edema and is unable to confirm any changes in weight. Worsening of dyspnea with exertion in this gentleman with a known abnormal cardiac stress test could be an anginal equivalent, even in the absence of chest symptoms. Increased abdominal girth with dyspnea could indicate a decompensation of his chronic liver disease. He has never been formally diagnosed with COPD but has a 40-pack-year smoking history, which certainly raises the possibility of obstructive lung disease with COPD exacerbation.

Management

Though referral to 911 and the ED would not be unreasonable, symptoms are subacute in nature, and patient's strong preference is to remain in his home. Given the wide differential diagnosis and lack of clinical assessment, simply doubling the patient's diuretic dosage without any additional information may have the potential to worsen rather than improve his condition. While an assessment from a skilled home health nurse would certainly be helpful, waiting until next week may result in the patient having further decompensation resulting in the need to go to the ED. Therefore, the best option is to try to gain additional information as soon as possible that can help in home-based assessment and management.

Outcome

Since Mr. S's home health nurse was not available until the following week, you referred him to the hospital's Community Paramedics to check vital signs including weight, draw labs including CBC, CMP, and pro-BNP and to obtain a 12-lead EKG [1]. You ordered a chest X-ray from a local portable imaging company and planned to visit the following day, when results of testing were available. On exam, patient's weight was stable as compared to the last 6 months; vital signs including oxygen saturations both at rest and with ambulation were within normal limits. His abdomen did appear distended, but there was no visible fluid wave, minimal peripheral edema, and no crackles on lung exam. However, he did appear quite short of breath with even minimal movement around his apartment and had diffuse mid to end expiratory wheezing on auscultation. Labs showed stable renal and hepatic function, no leukocytosis, and no elevation in BNP. CXR showed stable cardiac enlargement without pulmonary vascular congestion or focal infiltrate. You treated him for a COPD exacerbation with corticosteroids and azithromycin, which were delivered to his home from a local community pharmacy. You also ordered a nebulizer machine urgently through a durable medical equipment company for use with inhaled bronchodilators. You arranged with his home health agency to increase the frequency of skilled nursing visits to once daily for the period of 1 week, with follow-up physician home visits on days 1, 3, and 7. He responded well symptomatically and was ultimately started on a chronic inhaled corticosteroid in addition to his as-needed bronchodilators for long-term management of presumed chronic obstructive pulmonary disease.

Clinical Pearls and Pitfalls

- Many acute illnesses can be treated just as effectively at home as in the hospital and with lower costs and rates of complications [2–4].
- Community-based partners in care such as skilled home nursing agencies [5] and community paramedics can serve as physician extenders in the home to obtain additional clinical information for the treating physician and carry out provider orders for acute therapies.

- Portable imaging companies that provide services in skilled nursing facilities are also available to see homebound patients in private residences. Many communities have pharmacies and durable medical equipment companies who will deliver products to patients' homes. Having a working knowledge of what is available in your area is key to providing timely, home-based care for acute illnesses.

References

1. Abrashkin KA, Washko J, Zhang J, et al. Providing acute care at home: community paramedics enhance an advanced illness management program – preliminary data. J Am Geriatr Soc. 2016;64(12):2572–6.
2. Frick KD, Burton LC, Clark R, et al. Substitutive Hospital at Home for older persons: effects on costs. Am J Manag Care. 2009;15(1):49–56.
3. Leff B, Burton L, Mader S, et al. Hospital at Home: feasibility and outcomes of a program to provide hospital-level care at home for acutely ill older patients. Ann Intern Med. 2005;143:798–808.
4. Levine DM, Ouchi K, Blanchfield B, et al. Hospital-level care at home for acutely ill adults: a pilot randomized controlled trial. J Gen Intern Med. 2018;33(5):729–36.
5. Esslinger EE, Schade CP, Sun CK, et al. Exploratory analysis of the relationship between home health agency engagement in a national campaign and reduction in acute care hospitalization in US home care patients. J Eval Clin Pract. 2014;20(5):664–70.

Chapter 4
Dementia Behavior Management

Erin Zahradnik, Katherine Wang, Shahla Baharlou, and Jonathan Ripp

Case Study

You are going on a home visit to see Ms. J for worsening behavioral issues. Since assuming her care 6 months ago, you have visited twice and spoken on the phone with her daughter numerous times. She is 82 years old and has a history of coronary artery disease, hypertension, osteoarthritis, depression, constipation, and dementia. Her dementia history is described as starting about 8 years ago with mild short-term memory loss and word-finding difficulty. Since then, she has gradually required more assistance with shopping, cooking, and cleaning. Two years ago, she was found wandering in her neighborhood and sustained a fall while walking home. Since assuming her care, you have noted increasing deficits on serial cognitive

E. Zahradnik
University of Chicago, Chicago, IL, USA
e-mail: ezahradnik1@yoda.bsd.uchicago.edu

K. Wang (✉) · S. Baharlou · J. Ripp
Icahn School of Medicine at Mount Sinai, New York, NY, USA
e-mail: katherine.wang@mountsinai.org;
shahla.baharlou@mssm.edu; jonathan.ripp@mountsinai.org

© Springer Nature Switzerland AG 2020
J. L. Colburn et al. (eds.), *Home-Based Medical Care for Older Adults*, https://doi.org/10.1007/978-3-030-23483-6_4

testing and that she has had more difficulty managing most of her activities of daily living. She is now incontinent of urine, and your social worker recently worked with Pamela to increase the home attendant's hours to 6 hours a day, 5 days a week. The rest of the time, Ms. J is cared for by her daughter Pamela. She lives in a multigenerational home with her daughter, son-in-law, and two teenage grandchildren. For many years, she worked as a house cleaner while raising four children, three of whom now live out of state. Her spouse is deceased. She never smoked and drank alcohol only occasionally. Current medications include donepezil, amlodipine, lisinopril, sertraline, aspirin, senna, and acetaminophen.

In the last 3 weeks, Pamela reports that Ms. J has been sleeping more during the day and staying up several hours each night. She has been more confused, particularly in the afternoon, and has been increasingly resistant to allowing the home attendant to change her soiled diaper. She scratched the home attendant's arm during one such attempt. You, the visiting nurse, and your social worker have each spent time with Pamela and the home attendant counseling about non-pharmacologic approaches such as playing soft music, allowing the patient to scream during agitation episodes and reattempting to change her once she's calmed down. Now Pamela reports, "I'm exhausted. I can't take it anymore!" In the last few days, she has not slept and wonders if she needs to place her mother in a nursing home. You are being asked to urgently assess the patient and provide recommendations.

My Management

Assuming your examination and laboratory work do not reveal acute abnormality or infection, which could potentially cause these symptoms, which of the following would be the most appropriate next step?

A. Provide counseling for daughter and aides about trajectory of dementia.
B. Provide counseling as above and start antipsychotic.

C. Provide counseling as above and start a benzodiazepine.
D. Call 911 for emergency department evaluation, and consider nursing home placement.

Diagnosis and Assessment

Diagnosing dementia-related agitation is a diagnosis of exclusion; underlying factors that may contribute to acute delirium must be ruled out. Potentially reversible causes of agitation may include infection, metabolic disturbances, uremia, constipation/urinary retention, or medication-related side effect (e.g., corticosteroids, benzodiazepines, anticholinergics). Once it is firmly established that the agitation is secondary to dementia, providers and the interdisciplinary team can educate caregivers about non-pharmacologic interventions aimed at (1) providing education for both paid and unpaid caregivers, (2) reducing incidence of behaviors (e.g., identifying and minimizing triggers), and (3) responding to behaviors (e.g., providing reassurance and reorienting). Despite those efforts, escalation to pharmacotherapy may be necessary to protect the safety of the patient and caregivers and to allow for routine care.

In this case, the correct answer is (B)—provide counseling as above and start antipsychotic. While counseling is an essential part of management, at this point to allow for routine care (answer A), it would be incorrect to provide counseling only; you and your interdisciplinary team are convinced that the caregivers are maximizing behavioral approaches. Answer C is incorrect; a benzodiazepine should not be a first-line option for agitation. Finally, option D is incorrect as the underlying behavioral problems are likely to be exacerbated, rather than resolved, in an emergency room setting. For patients whose goals include remaining at home, the benefit of initiating of pharmacotherapy may outweigh the risk by ultimately allowing a patient to avoid placement in long-term care.

There is no widely accepted evidence of efficacy and safety for any pharmacotherapy for the treatment of behavioral problems in dementia. However, once behavioral interventions have been maximized, reversible causes of agitation are ruled out, and the safety of the patient/caregivers becomes a concern, providers can consider adding medication to the treatment algorithm.

Management

Caregivers must be trained to understand that behavioral problems may stem from a patient's unmet needs or limited ability to interpret or respond to a particular stimulus. Behavioral approaches encompass therapies ranging from general caregiver education and support, behavior-specific advice (e.g., identifying and reducing triggering stimuli), modification of environment (provision of music), to communication training (soft voice, avoidance of conflict, distraction) [1]. A home visit provider has the benefit of observing the patient in his or her home environment and may identify specific interventions that may be carried out, such as the orientation of the bed in relation to the door or window. Observation of caregivers performing routine care can also provide fodder for additional counseling; for instance, the provider may suggest that the home attendant perform bed baths with the patient partially covered at all times and using no-rinse products to reduce agitation.

Once the decision to add pharmacotherapy is made, providers should follow key geriatric principles of high-risk medication prescribing—start low, and go slow—while titrating to effective doses. Antipsychotics are typically the first class of medications utilized for severe dementia-related behavioral disturbances. Antipsychotics do convey an increased risk of death in patients with dementia (number needed to harm of 26–50 depending on medication) [2], especially those who have a significant cerebrovascular or cardiac history, so it is important to weigh the risks and benefits in terms of quality of life. While it is unclear which antipsychotic works best for particular behavioral symptoms, it can be helpful to choose one that has a favorable side effect profile. For example, a patient with sleep/wake reversal and subsequent nighttime agitation may benefit from a more sedating antipsychotic administered in the evening. Conversely, a patient with early afternoon agitation may require a less sedating antipsychotic given around lunchtime so as to specifically target the time-frame of aggressive behaviors. A patient with weight loss may do well with a medication that encourages appetite.

While there has been some recent suggestion in the literature of effectiveness of SSRIs in behavioral problems of dementia [3, 4], the most positive results have generally been in mild-moderate dementia with less severe agitation after several months of treatment [5]. Additionally, SSRIs are unlikely to provide the immediate effect desired for treatment of acute behavioral issues, so it may not be the first choice for a patient with more advanced dementia and care-impacting behaviors.

The use of anticonvulsants as mood stabilizers has even more limited evidence of efficacy in treating behavioral disturbances in dementia, and most of the positive findings are relegated to case studies [6].

Benzodiazepines and other sedatives should generally be reserved for last-line treatment, as they work by sedating the patient rather than directly mitigating behaviors and may precipitate paradoxical agitation in older patients.

Some early studies suggested a benefit in agitated dementia from anticholinesterase inhibitors such as donepezil and NMDA receptor antagonists like memantine. However, this was not borne out in later studies, so these medications are not recommended for behavioral problems alone [7].

If medications do not improve the patient's agitation, and it continues to impact her quality of life and put her and/or caregivers in danger, consider geriatric psychiatry referral. In some cases, short-term inpatient admission to a geriatric psychiatry unit for safe stabilization of a patient may be needed, with the aim to discharge back home.

Outcome

You and your social worker helped the patient's daughter devise some additional approaches to the patient's care. First, she found a trusted family member who could stay overnight several times a week to monitor the patient. Three times a week, the patient started attending a day program which then allowed for a reduction in the number of paid caregivers coming into the home; familiarity with her caregivers helped calm her considerably. After discussion of the risks and potential benefits, nightly quetiapine was initiated with some improvement in the sleep-wake cycle reversal. The behavioral modifications, along with the low-dose antipsychotic, brought her agitation to a manageable level for her daughter. At every visit, the use of medication for her behavior is re-evaluated.

Clinical Pearls and Pitfalls

- Behavioral approaches are the backbone of managing dementia-related behavioral issues (with or without pharmacotherapy) and may include modifying the environment in various ways (the built environment, caregivers, activities).
- Evidence for pharmacotherapy is limited, but medications may be an effective tool to allow patients to remain safely and comfortably at home; antipsychotics are typically the most common option with side effect profile determining which particular antipsychotic is used.
- Basic tenets: start low, go slow, titrate appropriately, and taper if able.
- With the support of your interdisciplinary team, obtaining information from and providing counseling to paid caregivers is often as important as supporting family or other unpaid caregivers.

References

1. Gitlin LN, Kales HC, Lyketsos CG. Managing behavioral symptoms in dementia using nonpharmacologic approaches: an overview. JAMA. 2012;308:2020–9.
2. Maust DT, Kim HM, Seyfried LS, et al. Antipsychotics, other psychotropics, and the risk of death in patients with dementia: number needed to harm. JAMA Psychiat. 2015;72:438–45.
3. Brodaty H. Antidepressant treatment in Alzheimer's disease. Lancet. 2011;378:375–6.
4. Porsteinsson AP, Drye LT, Pollock BG, et al. Effect of citalopram on agitation in Alzheimer disease: the CitAD randomized clinical trial. JAMA. 2014;311:682–91.
5. Schneider LS, Frangakis C, Drye LT, et al. Heterogeneity of treatment response to citalopram for patients with Alzheimer's disease with aggression or agitation: the CitAD randomized clinical trial. Am J Psychiatry. 2016;173:465–72.
6. Sink KM, Holden KF, Yaffe K. Pharmacological treatment of neuropsychiatric symptoms of dementia: a review of the evidence. JAMA. 2005;293(5):596.
7. Howard RJ, Juszczak E, Ballard CG, et al. Donepezil for the treatment of agitation in Alzheimer's disease. N Engl J Med. 2007;357:1382–92.

Chapter 5
Bacteriuria in a Patient with Incident Delirium

Thomas E. Finucane

Case Study

Ms. G is a 79-year-old retired investment banker who lives alone and is homebound with dense hemiplegia and some cognitive impairment. Three years ago, she suffered bilateral hemispheric strokes due to unsuspected atrial fibrillation. Her son calls you today because she seems unusually confused. She was fine last night although he had worked late, had forgone his customary visit, and had only spoken to her by phone. This morning she seems a bit withdrawn and upset and ate little breakfast. She refused or was unable to help him plan the lunch he usually prepared for her. Her expressive aphasia seemed worse, and he wondered if she was responding to internal stimuli because she was "brooding" and might have been mumbling to herself. A similar episode 10 months ago improved promptly with antibiotic treatment of a "urinary tract infection."

T. E. Finucane (✉)
Johns Hopkins University School of Medicine, Division of Geriatric Medicine & Gerontology, Baltimore, MD, USA
e-mail: tfinucan@jhmi.edu

© Springer Nature Switzerland AG 2020
J. L. Colburn et al. (eds.), *Home-Based Medical Care for Older Adults*, https://doi.org/10.1007/978-3-030-23483-6_5

Her medical history is generally benign other than the strokes, atrial fibrillation, hypertension, seasonal allergies, and chronic pain from a fall-related shoulder fracture. Her medications are apixaban, chlorthalidone, pregabalin, oxycodone, and as-needed antihistamine. She is a known dietary supplement enthusiast.

He says she seems well except for her behavior. Over the phone she is coherent but irritable, especially if her son offers any information. She denies any skin, gut, lung, or urinary symptoms. Urine is scant, turbid, and malodorous. The urine dipstick is positive for nitrites and leukocyte esterase.

My Management

Which of the following is the next best step?

A. Evaluate for other causes of mental status change, especially medication and supplement use, social factors, alcohol use, and trauma. Schedule the next available visit.
B. Prescribe an antibiotic for "UTI" and schedule the next available visit.
C. Prescribe quetiapine for sedation and schedule the next available visit.
D. Recommend a call to 911 for acute onset delirium.

Diagnosis and Assessment

Delirium can be an early signal of serious illness but is most often brief and self-limited. When persistent it requires careful evaluation. Belief in "UTI" as a cause of delirium often limits further evaluation and exposes patients to the risks and harms of unnecessary antibiotics.

The prevalence of asymptomatic bacteriuria, as determined by conventional urine cultures, in stable older women living independently is 11–16%, and for those in long-term care, it is 25–50%. (Corresponding figures for older men are 4–19% and 15–40%.) [1] The chance our patient, a vulnerable older woman at home, has bacteriuria by coincidence alone is likely in this range. The chance that she has bacteria in her urinary tract is 100%; a urinary tract microbiome has been identified using modern diagnostic techniques. Current clinical practice is based only on species that are detected using conventional urine cultures, a nineteenth-century technology. When we diagnose "UTI" and treat with antibiotics based on these cultures, and when we call the urine "sterile" when cultures are negative, we are simply agreeing to ignore any species that are difficult to identify.

There is no evidence that antibiotic treatment improves delirium outcomes in patients such as ours. In otherwise stable patients with incident delirium who have no urinary tract symptoms, expert guidance recommends against sending a urine culture, making a diagnosis of "UTI," or giving antibiotics [2, 3]. The Infectious Disease Society of America's 2019 Clinical Practice Guideline update says, "In older patients with functional and/or cognitive impairment with bacteriuria and delirium (acute mental status change, confusion) and without local genitourinary symptoms or other systemic signs of infection (eg, fever or hemodynamic instability), we recommend assessment for other causes and careful observation rather than antimicrobial treatment." [4].

Antipsychotic use in older patients carries lethal risk and is best reserved for psychotic symptoms. In this case our goal would be sedation, which could mask persistent delirium and delay a thorough evaluation.

Emergency rooms and hospitals can worsen delirium. Because delirium can be an early signal of catastrophic illness, prompt antibiotic treatment may be lifesaving in unstable patients. For our patient, who does not seem seriously ill, the harms of hospitalization and of antibiotic or antipsychotic treatment tilt the risk/benefit equation toward careful evaluation and anxious observation.

Management

Two challenges to management await. To persuade the son to accept watchful waiting may be difficult, especially since his mother has previously improved with antibiotics for a "UTI" in a similar situation. Suggest that the prior episode would likely have cleared even if antibiotics had not been given. (Patient and family may be remarkably certain of causality when self-limited illness improves with antibiotic treatment.) Present the lack of evidence of benefit and clear evidence of harms, and review the expert advice against treatment. Discuss the high, in fact universal, prevalence of bacteriuria. But reason is not a uniformly successful tool. If antibiotics are socially necessary (e.g., "I'll take her to the ED if you won't treat her"), a fallback strategy is to obtain a urine culture and start treatment. Stop treatment if the culture is negative (use this as an opportunity to educate the son). If the culture is positive, complete a short course. A second challenge is to arrange adequate monitoring of the situation. The more vulnerable she is, the more intense the necessary monitoring. And if she worsens or, after a few days, fails to improve, more intensive investigation may be required.

Outcome

The patient improved within a day with no explanation of the confusion's cause or resolution. Her home nurse mentioned that increased job responsibilities were taking up progressively more of the son's time and that the patient sometimes expressed her resentment nonverbally. The patient acknowledged a recent dietary supplement purchase on Amazon unbeknownst to her son, but only after she had discarded the product. She declined your suggestion to manage her oxycodone, pregabalin, antihistamines, and supplements more judiciously.

Clinical Pearls and Pitfalls

- Calling asymptomatic bacteriuria a "UTI" and treating it as the cause of delirium is a major cause of antibiotic overuse.
- Delirium can be a harbinger of catastrophe but is usually self-limited.

- Asymptomatic bacteriuria is highly prevalent in frail older adults. With modern diagnostic techniques, a ubiquitous urinary microbiome is seen.
- No evidence shows that antibiotic treatment of bacteriuria in an otherwise well patient with incident delirium will improve delirium outcomes.

References

1. Nicolle LE, Bradley S, Colgan R, et al. Infectious Diseases Society of America guidelines for the diagnosis and treatment of asymptomatic bacteriuria in adults. Clin Infect Dis. 2005;40(5):643–54.
2. Finucane TE. "Urinary tract infection" – requiem for a heavyweight. J Am Geriatr Soc. 2017;65(8):1650–5.
3. McKenzie R, Stewart MT, Bellantoni MF, Finucane TE. Bacteriuria in individuals who become delirious. Am J Med. 2014;127(4):255–7.
4. Nicolle LE, Gupta K, Bradley SF, Colgan R, DeMuri GP, Drekonja D, Eckert LO, Geerlings SE, Köves B, Hooton TM, Juthani-Mehta M, Knight SL, Saint S, Schaeffer AJ, Trautner B, Wullt B, Siemieniuk R. Clinical practice guideline for the management of asymptomatic bacteriuria: 2019 update by the Infectious Diseases Society of Americaa. Clin Infect Dis. 2019. pii: ciy1121. https://doi.org/10.1093/cid/ciy1121.

Chapter 6
Caregiver Burden

Mia Yang and Rachel Zimmer

Case Study

Today you are seeing Mr. A, an 83-year-old man with Alzheimer's dementia who is a new patient to the home-based primary care (HBPC) program. He lives with his wife, Mrs. A, who has been caring for him over the last several years as his cognition has declined. Mr. A has gradually required more assistance with bathing and toileting and has had several falls over the past 6 months. Mrs. A is 80 years old and has her own health problems to manage as well. They do not have any children or family nearby to help them. When you walk into the house, you notice a strong odor of urine. The one-story house is cluttered. You open the fridge and there is little to no food. There are some opened cans of chicken noodle soup sitting in the sink.

Mrs. A states that their marriage before Mr. A's diagnosis of Alzheimer's disease has always been "rocky." Since his dementia has progressed, she has felt more resentful of the

M. Yang (✉) · R. Zimmer
Wake Forest School of Medicine, Winston Salem, NC, USA
e-mail: miyang@wakehealth.edu

© Springer Nature Switzerland AG 2020
J. L. Colburn et al. (eds.), *Home-Based Medical Care for Older Adults*, https://doi.org/10.1007/978-3-030-23483-6_6

amount of time and care that he requires. She has no one to help her and feels like her own retirement has "gone to waste" by caring for him. She admits that sometimes she cannot get Mr. A to the bathroom on time, so she puts him in a diaper as much as possible. His personality has become more difficult as his memory has declined. Now he is irritable, stubborn, and resistant to help. She feels as if she would be "giving up" if she were to place him in a facility. They are financially limited, and she does not have enough money to buy food and medications for both of them. His medication list includes fluticasone/salmeterol, albuterol nebulizer, metoprolol succinate, amlodipine, levothyroxine, donepezil, memantine, aspirin, omeprazole, atorvastatin, trazodone, tamsulosin, and hydrocodone-acetaminophen. Their income together is too high to be eligible for Medicaid, and they cannot afford to hire in-home help.

My Management

Which of the following should be your next step?

A. File a report with Adult Protective Services
B. Refer to social worker affiliated with home health agency
C. Assess for care partner burden with a validated scale
D. Refer for home health nursing services

Diagnosis and Assessment

Assessing care partner burden can be a complex assessment because it involves knowledge of care partner's psychological symptoms, demands that illness has imposed on them, and the care partner's predisposition to having negative or positive experiences during caregiving. Often care partners with high burden will suffer in silence instead of reaching out for resources on their own. Many times, a care partner needs guidance on how to access and obtain resources.

Identifying care partner burden with a validated tool is the first step to a person-centered approach to managing the symptoms of burden [1, 2]. The Zarit Burden Interview (ZBI) measures a care partner's perceived burden of providing care on a 5-point Likert scale, ranging from a total score of 0–88, with higher scores indicating greater burden. Domains of burden include time, level of stress, anger, guilt, health, financial, and sense of control.

Although other choices listed above may be appropriate in this case, the assessment of care partner's burden is the best first choice, as it provides a framework for targeting the items considered most burdensome to the care partner. For example, if the care partner is most distressed by financial limitations, then simplifying medications and referral to Meals on Wheels may be appropriate. A referral to Adult Protective Services without gathering more information and determining need may alienate the care partner and damage the provider-patient-care partner relationship. Unless the patient has an existing home health agency involved with their care, the provider cannot open a new home health case with a social worker referral. A referral for home health nursing would be helpful if the care partner identified a need that required the skills of a nurse to address such as wound care or medication management.

Management

After assessing care partner burden with a validated tool such as the ZBI, a provider and interdisciplinary team should help to develop targeted and individualized interventions. Research suggests that care partners should receive education and support early in the disease process to help prepare for the future and that the provider should offer anticipatory guidance at regular intervals related to the disease progression [3, 4]. Providers should ensure that interventions are culturally sensitive and that the care partner is involved in the planning of any interventions [3, 5]. Psychotherapy, in the form of cognitive behavioral therapy, and psychoeducational sessions are recommended interventions that can help a care partner cope with his or her role in caregiving [5–7]. These interventions assist care partners in the development of skills that help to problem-solve and promote coping behaviors [5]. It is especially important to ensure that education, information, and support programs are available to the care partner in times of transition [4]. Technology is one tool to connect to care partners who cannot easily leave the home or who might be interested in online support programs.

Community Resources

The care of individuals with dementia and their care partners requires support from multiple avenues due to the disease's complexity and significant time required of the care partner. Many times, care partners feel alone in their role and as a result may begin to feel resentment and guilt. The Alzheimer's Association provides access to telephonic support groups and a variety of caregiver resources online. These resources can also be printed for Mrs. A. if she does not have access to a computer. Educating Mrs. A about how to address Mr. A's behaviors can give her the tools that she needs to utilize proven strategies and make her feel more confident in her caregiving abilities. Often, financial stress plays a role in care partner burden, and by connecting Mrs. A to a social worker, the provider can connect Mrs. A to resources that she might not already be aware of to help with their financial situation. For example, Meals on Wheels can help to supplement meals for a family who is having difficulty paying for or accessing food.

Outcome

You ask Mrs. A to complete the ZBI while you are examining Mr. A. She scores 60 points, which indicates severe caregiver burden. Specifically she checks off "nearly always" to the following: "Do you feel angry when you are around your relative?", "Do you feel your health has suffered because of your involvement with your relative?","Do you wish you could leave the care of your relative to someone else?", and "Do you feel that you have lost control of your life since your relative's illness?"

You work with Mrs. A to prioritize both her and Mr. A's needs. She reports that she feels particularly stressed about not having access to food because of the cost of their medications. She also feels very alone in her role as a care partner. After your discussion with her, you:

1. Educate Mrs. A on her husband's dementia behaviors and provide some coping strategies for "hot button" behaviors.
2. Acknowledge Mrs. A's emotions of guilt, shame, resentment, and anger, and work with her to plan for the future.
3. Connect them to your HBPC social worker or the local senior services agency.
4. Refer Mrs. A to an Alzheimer's disease support group that provides telephone access for care partners unable to join in person.
5. Set up Meals on Wheels for meal supplementation.
6. Switch medications to generics, and reduce polypharmacy for Mr. A so that cost of medications is cheaper.

Clinical Pearls and Pitfalls

- Caregiver burden can produce significant physical and mental health problems for individuals [3].
- It is helpful to systematically assess caregiver burden with a valid scale such as the Zarit Burden Interview to help identify distress and monitor effectiveness of interventions [1, 2].
- A person-centered approach should be applied when providing options for caregiver or care partner support [4, 5, 7].
- Evidence shows that psychotherapy, specifically cognitive behavioral therapy, and psychoeducation interventions

that combine education and counseling are the most likely interventions to improve symptoms of caregiver burden [5–7].

References

1. Zarit SH, Reever KE, Bach-Peterson J. Relatives of the impaired elderly: correlates of feelings of burden. Gerontologist. 2010;20(6):649–55.. Available for individual clinician download: https://eprovide.mapi-trust.org/instruments/zarit-burden-interview
2. Seng B, Luo N, Ng W, et al. Validity and reliability of the Zarit Burden interview in assessing caregiver burden. Ann Acad Med Singap. 2010;39(10):758–63.
3. McCabe M, You E, Tatangelo G. Hearing their voice: a systematic review of dementia family caregivers' needs. Gerontologist. 2016;56(5):e70–88.
4. Whitlatch CJ, Orsulic-Jeras S. Meeting the informational, educational, and psychosocial support needs of persons living with dementia and their family caregivers. The Gerontologist. 2018;58(S1):S58–73.
5. Parker D, Mills S, Abbey J. Effectiveness of interventions that assist caregivers to support people with dementia living in the community: a systematic review. Int J Evid Based Healthcare. 2008;6:137–72.
6. Gilhooly KJ, Gilhooly ML, Sullivan MP, et al. A meta-review of stress, coping, and interventions in dementia and dementia caregiving. BMC Geriatr. 2016;16:106.
7. Pinquart M, Sorenson S. Helping caregivers of persons with dementia: which interventions work and how large are their effects? Int Psychogeriatric. 2006;18:577–95.

Chapter 7
Elder Abuse and Neglect

Ania Wajnberg, Sarah Koppel, and Fay Kahan

Case Study

Mr. B is a 70-year-old man whom you are seeing today at home with your team social worker for a house call. He has multiple sclerosis and requires assistance to transfer from his bed to his wheelchair. Mr. B has Medicaid and 24-hour paid help at home. His sister helps to manage his finances. The social worker received a phone call from Mr. B's paid caregiver that Mr. B cannot pay his rent, as he currently has no money in his account. The social worker has been working with the patient for several years and suspects that patient's sister has been using his money to pay some of her own bills. You and the social worker are making a house call together to discuss your concerns with Mr. B and to explore options. You assess capacity and feel that Mr. B has capacity to make financial decisions. He says he named his sister as his financial power of attorney since he is unable to leave his home

A. Wajnberg
Icahn School of Medicine at Mount Sinai, New York, NY, USA

S. Koppel (✉) · F. Kahan
Mount Sinai Health System, New York, NY, USA
e-mail: sarah.koppel@mountsinai.org

© Springer Nature Switzerland AG 2020   41
J. L. Colburn et al. (eds.), *Home-Based Medical Care for Older Adults*, https://doi.org/10.1007/978-3-030-23483-6_7

and gets overwhelmed managing his financial issues and his health issues. You ask the patient to describe what he knows about his finances, and he says this is not the first time his sister has used his money for other family member needs and says he will talk with her. The social worker recommends making an Adult Protective Services (APS) referral and filing a police report to recoup the money. Mr. B declines initially as he says that he knows his sister is going through a hard time and he does not want to get her in trouble so will say that he agreed to lend her the money, but then he starts receiving creditor mail for multiple different agencies so agrees to an APS assessment. He does not want the social worker to file a police report, as he says he will not press charges against his sister.

My Management

Which of the following is the next best step in management?

A. Meet with team, patient, and family.
B. Increase home care.
C. Call law enforcement.
D. Pursue guardianship.

Diagnosis and Assessment

In recent years, elder abuse has received more attention in medical and social screenings, but definitions of what constitutes abuse or neglect can vary, and there is no consensus on screening criteria in the literature or in practical use. The Centers for Disease Control and Prevention (CDC) defines abuse as "intentional act or failure to act by a caregiver or another person in a relationship involving an expectation of trust that causes or creates a serious risk of harm to an older adult" [1]. There are five widely accepted types of elder abuse: physical, emotional/psychological, sexual, neglect, and financial abuse.

National studies using self-report data have estimated the prevalence of elder abuse between 8 and 10%, and this is likely an underestimate, as abuse often goes unreported and unrecognized [2–4]. It has been reported that older women are more likely to be victims of abuse than men [4]. Living with one or more other people, having lower income, isolation, cognitive deficits, behavioral health issues, and lack of social supports have all been associated with higher likelihood of all types of elder abuse. Although no studies on elder abuse focus on the homebound population specifically, given that people who are homebound often rely on caregivers to stay in the community, may be isolated due to poor functional status, and may have cognitive impairment, elder abuse is important to consider in the homebound population. Along with the ethical and home safety issues affected when one suspects elder abuse, providers should be aware that elder abuse has been shown to be an independent risk factor for hospitalization, nursing home placement, and even death [5, 6].

Given the relatively high prevalence of elder abuse and the high percentage of homebound patients who are at risk for elder abuse, home-based primary care providers and caregivers (both formal and informal) need education on how to screen, assess, identify, and handle suspicions of elder abuse. Patients with multiple medical problems and cognitive impairment may find it difficult or impossible to report abuse themselves, and providers may identify issues that trigger further investigation into home safety. These triggers may include physical signs of abuse, such as bruises, lacerations, abrasions, fractures, rashes, or burns, particularly if they take place without a clear explanation. Sexually transmitted infections (STIs) in homebound patients should be considered in the context of cognitive function and ability to consent to sexual activity. If patients are noted to have poor personal hygiene, inadequate cleaning or diaper changing, or dehydration or malnutrition, one should assess for neglect. A change in ability to pay for food, medical care, medications, and durable medical equipment or a change to adherence to a prior medical regimen might indicate financial abuse. In all cases, these issues can be multifactorial, benign, or related to factors other than abuse, but abuse must be considered and evaluated. Providers who suspect abuse in the home setting should work with an interdisciplinary team and ideally a social worker or other mental health professional with expertise in this area. If a home-based primary care team does not have a social worker or mental health professional, partnerships with nursing or social service agencies in the community might be able to help with a full assessment and plan. Various tools are available to screen for abuse, including the Elder Abuse Suspicion Index (EASI) [7] and the Vulnerability to Abuse Screening Scale (VASS) [8]. It is important to consider that there may be more than one type of abuse happening, and all five areas should be assessed when abuse is suspected.

Management

Initially, the suspicion for abuse in Mr. B's situation came from a phone call from the paid personal caregiver. Group discussion by the health-care team, including the social worker, nurse, physician, and administrative staff, revealed several prior phone calls related to concerns regarding unexplained bruises on Mr. B and missed visits by the sister after agreements to meet providers in the home. For Mr. B, the team's social worker began frequent and regular home visits in order to engage the patient in the assessment process and used validated tools to screen for all five areas of abuse – physical, emotional/psychological, sexual, neglect, and financial. Engagement of a family member or suspected abuser may be necessary to address the abuse suspicion and potential solutions. For Mr. B, you arranged a family meeting including the patient, his sister, and the entire medical team, to discuss concerns and next steps. His sister initially said she did not take his money without his permission, but the team was able to share concerns that Mr. B had not given permission and was not able to meet his own care needs since the money had been displaced to other family members' needs. Family members were willing to consider alternative options, and the patient and medical team did not feel there was a need to put an order of protection in place. You referred the patient to Adult Protective Services for support and ongoing assessment. The team continued to work with the patient to implement these steps and potentially to select a new financial power of attorney due to his sister's ongoing financial challenges and difficulty managing Mr. B's financial needs in accordance with his needs and wishes.

Outcome

You and the social worker visited Mr. B several times to develop trust and further engage him. As a result, he agreed to work with Adult Protective Services (APS) to consider alternative care arrangements. In collaboration with APS, you and your team recommended that he consider selecting a new financial power of attorney to ensure that he is able to pay his bills to stay in his apartment. He asked another sibling who was willing to assist with financial matters. APS communicated with the bank to monitor and address any unexpected withdrawals. You and the team social worker continued to assess at each visit for other forms of abuse and neglect. You also conducted cognitive testing to confirm capacity and decision-making abilities.

It is important to note that patients do not need guardianship if they are able to make their own financial decisions, but a financial power of attorney may be helpful if the patient wishes to have additional protection against elder abuse and neglect, assistance with bills, or is having difficulty with managing finances. A financial power of attorney can then assist with finances while still involving the patient with financial decision-making. They do not need to involve the patient, however. When a patient no longer has capacity to make financial decisions, then a representative payee or guardian could be appointed.

Clinical Pearls and Pitfalls

- Elder abuse is often undetected and underreported in the homebound population. It is important that home-based providers understand the signs of abuse and neglect and assess for it if there are signs or concerns.
- Female gender, living with others, lower socioeconomic status, isolation, cognitive deficits, and lack of social supports are all associated with a higher risk of elder abuse.
- Homebound patients may be at a higher risk of abuse and non-reporting due to isolation and dependence on family to remain in the community.
- Interdisciplinary team communication and collaboration is essential for assessment and treatment of patients who are experiencing elder abuse.

References

1. Centers for Disease Control, National Center for Injury Prevention and Control, Division of Violence Prevention. Elder abuse surveillance: uniform definitions and recommended core data elements. Atlanta: U.S. Department of Health and Human Services; 2016. https://www.cdc.gov/violenceprevention/pdf/ea_book_revised_2016.pdf. Accessed 11 Apr 2019.
2. Burnes D, Pillemer K, Caccamise PL, et al. Prevalence of and risk factors for elder abuse and neglect in the community: a population-based study. J Am Geriatr Soc. 2015;63:1906–12.
3. Acierno R, Hernandez MA, Amstadter AB, et al. Prevalence and correlates of emotional, physical, sexual, and financial abuse and potential neglect in the United States: the National Elder Mistreatment Study. Am J Public Health. 2010;100:292–7.
4. Laumann EO, Leitsch SA, Waite LJ. Elder mistreatment in the United States: prevalence estimates from a nationally representative study. J Gerontol B Psychol Sci Soc Sci. 2008;63:S248–54.
5. Murphy K, Waa S, Jaffer H, et al. A literature review of findings in physical elder abuse. Can Assoc Radiol J. 2013;64:10–4.
6. Gibbs L, Mosqueda L. Elder abuse: a medical perspective. Aging Health. 2010;6:739–47.

7. Yaffe MJ, Wolfson C, Lithwick M, Weiss D. Development and validation of a tool to improve physician identification of elder abuse: the Elder Abuse Suspicion Index (EASI). J Elder Abuse Negl. 2008;20(3):276–300.
8. Schofield MJ, Mishra G. Validity of self report screening scale for elder abuse. The Gerontologist. 2003;43(1):110–20.

Chapter 8
Management of Frequent Falls

Mattan Schuchman and Joseph Graziano

Case Study

Mr. T returned home last week after a 3-day hospitalization for pneumonia. You are conducting a follow-up house call. Mr. T is an 81-year-old retired carpenter who is homebound due to osteoarthritis of his knees and hips. He has diabetes, hypertension, and lung cancer in complete remission after chemotherapy. Before the hospitalization, he had occasional falls, about once a month, and never sustained serious injury. Since returning home, Mr. T has fallen daily—mostly in his bedroom—and he has been too nervous to attempt bathing. He does not understand why he is falling more frequently. He reports that he has increased dyspnea on exertion and feels weaker. He does not lose consciousness, experience palpitations, have jerking movements, or have dizzy spells prior to his falls. Rather, he

M. Schuchman (✉)
Johns Hopkins University School of Medicine, Baltimore, MD, USA
e-mail: mattan@jhmi.edu

J. Graziano
Johns Hopkins Home Care Group, Baltimore, MD, USA

© Springer Nature Switzerland AG 2020   49
J. L. Colburn et al. (eds.), *Home-Based Medical Care for Older Adults*, https://doi.org/10.1007/978-3-030-23483-6_8

describes the falls as "my legs just give out." He reports varying levels of pain in his knees and hips with mobility and activities of daily living (ADLs). Mr. T is completing a 7-day course of oral antibiotics for pneumonia; his other medications were not changed in the hospital. On your examination, Mr. T is normotensive and has no change in heart rate or blood pressure between lying, sitting, and standing. He has multiple balance, range of motion, and strength deficits. He cannot stand from a seated position without using his upper extremities and "plops" in his chair when sitting down. Gait is slow with a wide base of support, and he cannot maintain balance with his eyes closed. Sensory testing reveals poor sensation to light touch in his feet. Mr. T lives in a single floor setup with four steps and a railing leading to the entrance. The lighting is dim. He has a walker but finds it difficult to use because the arrangement of furniture and personal possessions leaves narrow walkways.

My Management

What is your next step?

A. Refer to a skilled nursing facility for inpatient rehabilitation.
B. Discontinue all medications that could contribute to falls.
C. Assess mobility, strength, and balance in the home environment and consult physical therapy.
D. Refer to cardiology for an event monitor.
E. Obtain brain imaging as well as blood levels including BMP, CBC, and vitamin D.

The correct answer is: C

Diagnosis and Assessment

You have two issues to unravel in this case: the cause for falls at baseline and the recent increase in fall frequency. Maintaining balance is a complex skill that requires the integration of tactile, visual, proprioceptive, and vestibular sensation with moment-to-moment fine and gross motor adjustments. The ability to maintain balance diminishes in older adults due to sensory losses and decreased muscle strength and control. Mr. T's history provides important clues to the underlying diagnosis and next steps in management.

Mr. T has no focal neurologic deficits or seizure-like symptoms, so brain imaging is not necessary. Blood testing is unlikely to reveal a cause for falls. Vitamin D deficiency, if present, cannot account for Mr. T's recent increased falling; evidence does not support vitamin D supplementation to prevent falls in a community-dwelling adult [1]. Cardiac arrhythmia or carotid sinus hypersensitivity, though concerning, is also less likely, as Mr. T can describe his legs faltering and does not experience syncope or palpitations. An event monitor is thus not the appropriate next step. Medications are a frequent contributor to falls, but stopping all medications associated with falls without carefully weighing the risks and benefits of each would be inappropriate. Inpatient rehabilitation at a subacute facility may be helpful in cases when a person cannot safely remain at home or requires daily treatments with a physical therapist. However, for most homebound individuals, such as Mr. T, a provider can adequately assess and treat falls in the home with help from a home health physical therapist.

Your evaluation should start with a thorough examination and assessment of Mr. T's mobility, strength, and balance in the home environment. Mr. T's decrease in balance at baseline most likely resulted from his medical conditions, which include pain and limited range of motion (ROM) from osteoarthritis and neuropathy from diabetes and prior chemotherapy. Risk factors in his home environment, such as dim lighting and trip hazards, contributed to the baseline risk. After his hospitalization, Mr. T's falls frequency increased due to weakness from a recent bedrest, decreased exercise tolerance from pneumonia, and a new fear of falling.

Management

The American Geriatrics Society (AGS) and Centers for Disease Control and Prevention (CDC) recommend a multifactorial intervention for reducing frequent falls [2, 3]. The first step in this intervention is the completion of a risk assessment, which will help identify risk factors for falls that may be modifiable. Key components of the assessment include physical assessment, environmental assessment, and medication review. This chapter will focus on the physical assessment and management; for a discussion of home assessment and medication review, see Chaps. 9 and 16, respectively.

In a homebound patient who has frequent falls, the provider should pay particular attention to physical findings that may be amenable to adaptations or treatments to reduce falls. These findings may include balance, orthostatic vitals, cognition, sensation, muscle weakness, range of motion (ROM), footwear, eyewear, assistive devices, and pain levels. Home-based exercise programs (HEPs) are an evidence-based approach to reduce the risk of falls that result from weakness, ROM, or balance problems, as in Mr. T's case [4]. The physical assessment helps tailor the exercise and balance intervention to the individual's needs. Collaboration with a physical therapist is invaluable for completing a full physical assessment and for creating and implementing the treatment plan in the home. A complete HEP will include training on ROM, balance, strength, and gait; a therapist may work with a patient on each of these domains concurrently. A therapist will increase the challenge and complexity of the exercises as the patient regains functional ability or will adapt exercises to create realistic and achievable goals (see Chap. 15).

Functional ROM for the ankles, knees, and hips is key to fall prevention. The first goal for Mr. T is therefore to increase active and passive ROM of the lower extremities. Most patients have adequate hip and knee flexion but lack sufficient extension to maintain stability. Hip extension can be evaluated by having Mr. T hold a walker for support and kick back as far as possible without flexing at the hips or low back. If Mr. T can get close to a natural posture (0 degrees of hip extension), it will facilitate his ability to walk without a walker and to reach above his head. Mr. T must also develop adequate ROM of the ankles in order to remain balanced and steady while extending his upper extremities. A provider can assess ankle dorsiflexion (DF) and plantarflexion (PF) while a patient is lying down or by asking them to stand on their toes and then rock back on their heels while holding on to a stable object for support. Adequate active ROM for most activities and gait is 10–15 degrees of DF and 25–30 degrees of PF.

Sufficient lower extremity (LE) and core strength is required to maintain stability while walking or transferring from sit to stand. Gluteus medius strength is important for stability while walking and is commonly lacking in older adults. A HEP for gluteus medius strengthening could begin with side-lying hip exercises, such as bent-knee leg lifts, and progress to side-lying straight leg raises or standing hip abduction exercises (kicking out to the side) with and without elastic resistance. Because Mr. T is ambulatory, a therapist may ask Mr. T to stand with upper extremity (UE) support while performing LE exercises to strengthen his ankles, hips, and knees (i.e., heel and toe lifts, small knee bends, marching in place, kicking backward) and gradually decrease the UE support to increase the load on his LE and core muscles.

As strength and ROM improve, Mr. T can work on balance exercises. Balance exercises should begin with stationary (static) postures using a wide base of support, first with eyes open and eventually with eyes closed. Mr. T might then progress to a narrow-based standing position; to tandem stance (feet positioned in a straight line); and to standing on one leg, first with and then perhaps without UE support. Functional applications—such as reaching with arms extended above the head and below the knees and while holding an appropriate amount of weight—will further challenge his dynamic balance. Completing dynamic balance exercises on varied standing surfaces (i.e., mats, carpet, foam pads, balance boards, etc.) will prepare Mr. T for the demands of most of his functional activities in the home.

Finally, gait training to gradually increase walking duration and speed will help improve Mr. T's endurance and tolerance for safe ambulation. Improved gait mechanics may also result in reduced pain levels. Due to patterns Mr. T may have developed with his gait, extra time may be required for him to adopt optimal gait mechanics. For patients with dyspnea, appropriate pacing, breathing strategies, and pauses for recovery periods are essential to improve oxygenation levels and reduce dyspnea and fatigue. If warranted for safe ambulation, training on the use of any appropriate assistive device is an important component of treatment.

Outcome

By your 1-month follow-up with Mr. T, he has been seeing the physical therapist two to three times a week and has progressed nicely through his HEP. His daughter learned the exercises and agreed to help him continue them after home physical therapy is completed. Mr. T also received an evaluation from the home health occupational therapist. The occupational therapist showed Mr. T new strategies for safely completing household activities, such as using the commode and shower and cooking. In addition, Mr. T embraced some of the safety recommendations from the physical and occupational therapists. Mr. T changed his bifocals into single-lens glasses, which helped him avoid obstacles on the floor. He bought a well-fitting pair of tennis shoes with a nonslip sole. His daughter, who is a carpenter like her father, installed brighter lighting and a strategic grab bar in the shower. Mr. T agreed to move some, though not all, of his beloved possessions into boxes, thereby clearing wider walkways and removing trip hazards. He started scheduled acetaminophen, which improved his arthritis pain. He now uses a shower chair to reduce risk of slipping in the shower, and the occupational therapist taught him how to safely transfer to and from the shower chair. His dyspnea on exertion returned to baseline as the pneumonia cleared. Mr. T reports that he still occasionally loses his balance, but his rate of falling returned to what it was before his pneumonia. Mr. T tells you that he is no longer afraid of falling and has started bathing independently again.

Clinical Pearls and Pitfalls

1. Homebound older adults are at an elevated risk for falls. Evaluation of fall history is an important component of every home assessment and can help determine the cause of and treatment for falls.
2. Assessing gait, balance, and mobility within the lived environment, in collaboration with home health physical and occupational therapists, is the first step for management of homebound patients who have fallen or nearly fallen.
3. A multifactorial intervention, including a tailored home exercise program for balance, strength, and safety, can reduce the frequency of future falls.

References

1. Guirguis-Blake JM, Michael YL, Perdue LA, et al. Interventions to prevent falls in older adults: updated evidence report and systematic review for the US preventive services task force. JAMA. 2019;319:1705–16.
2. Centers for Disease Control and Prevention. STEADI – older adult fall prevention 2017. Atlanta: U.S. Department of Health & Human Services; 2017. https://www.cdc.gov/steadi/index.html. Accessed 8 Oct 2018.
3. Panel on Prevention of Falls in Older Persons, American Geriatrics Society and British Geriatrics Society. Summary of the updated American Geriatrics Society/British Geriatrics Society clinical practice guideline for prevention of falls in older persons. J Am Geriatr Soc. 2011;59:148–57.
4. Gillespie LD, Robertson MC, Gillespie WJ, et al. Interventions for preventing falls in older people living in the community. Cochrane Database Syst Rev. 2012;9:CD007146.

Chapter 9
Home Assessments—Improving Patients' Capacity for Self-Management

Monika Robinson and Sarah L. Szanton

Case Study

You arrive at Ms. D's home, an 82-year-old woman with lumbar stenosis and multiple recurrent hospitalizations for exacerbations of heart failure. She demonstrates increased shortness of breath, antalgic gait, and difficulty locking the door. You assess her understanding of preventive measures she can take to avoid another exacerbation, such as weighing herself daily and taking her medication. After this, you inquire if she has been taking her medication and weighing herself daily. She thinks she has taken the medication but isn't certain if she has taken it as prescribed. She is unable to tell which pills she's taken and has a hard time reading the labels. Her medications are not accurately filled in her daily pill box.

M. Robinson (✉)
Department of Occupational Therapy, Midwestern University, Downers Grove, IL, USA
e-mail: mrobin@midwestern.edu

S. L. Szanton
John Hopkins School of Nursing, Baltimore, MD, USA
e-mail: sszanto1@jhu.edu

© Springer Nature Switzerland AG 2020
J. L. Colburn et al. (eds.), *Home-Based Medical Care for Older Adults*, https://doi.org/10.1007/978-3-030-23483-6_9

She doesn't like taking the diuretic because sitting on the toilet hurts her back, so she does it as little as possible. She hasn't gotten on the scale on the second floor. Ms. D reports it has been increasingly difficult to do what she needs to do to take care of herself at home because of low back pain radiating along her left leg, making it difficult for her to stand, walk, or get up from a seated position. Her limited mobility around the home makes it impossible for her to prepare any meals unless they are frozen or canned foods that she can quickly microwave. She states she feels as if this is all too much for her and appears to be despondent about her current health condition and functional abilities.

My Management

Which of the following is the next best step in management?

A. Prescribe an anti-inflammatory for the pain due to lumbar stenosis.
B. Focus on reinforcing patient's adherence to heart failure medication regimen for symptom management.
C. Assess patient's safety and functional independence within the home.
D. Perform Mini-Mental State Exam (MMSE).

Diagnosis and Assessment

Chronic conditions such as heart failure frequently have associated conditions such as reduced cognition and visual loss [1, 2]. How patients and their primary care providers medically manage the chronic conditions is contingent upon how well the patient functions within their home environment. The patient may be experiencing many obstacles that impede their ability to effectively self-manage their chronic conditions. These barriers may exist within the patient's home environment rather than within the patient exclusively.

An effective self-management plan goes beyond the patient's medical condition or impairments and instead needs to incorporate how the patient's impairments impact their ability to function within their home. An assessment of the home environment may reveal many barriers, such as insufficient lighting, inaccessible entryways, low seating heights, and improper furniture placement. These environmental barriers could lead to an inability to obtain necessary household items, difficulty performing essential daily self-care tasks, and poor adherence with nutritional and medication guidelines resulting in an exacerbation of the patient's chronic conditions. Prescribing an anti-inflammatory, reinforcing adherence, and performing a Mini-Mental State Exam will not get to the root of the self-management problem, and the anti-inflammatory may impair her kidney function, leading to additional problems. Assessing how the patient interfaces in the home to ensure the patient is able to perform self-care/management, activities of daily living (ADLs), and instrumental activities of daily living (IADLs) is necessary and has been proven to be efficacious in improving management of chronic conditions [3–5].

Management

Home-based interventions that address the mismatch between the patient's abilities and the home environment can optimize an older adult's ability to safely age in place [6]. A multidisciplinary preventive approach providing free assistive devices, adaptive techniques from an occupational therapist (OT), home modifications completed by a handyman, and skill building regarding medication and symptom management from a registered nurse (RN) has shown significant healthcare cost savings for older adults with disability [7]. Focusing on a patient's self-identified functional goals, cognitive and low vision strategies using adaptive techniques and task-specific exercises improves older adults' performance with ADLs and IADLs [6–8].

Outcome

In Ms. D's case, you note that she is unable to read nutrition labels or see which medications she has taken because of her low vision. She cannot adhere to her dietary restrictions due to the limited variety of food she can prepare. She cannot access her scale on the second floor due to difficulty climbing stairs. You observe her flat affect and possible depression and provide a referral for a home assessment through a multidisciplinary team. An OT addresses her functional performance with ADL and IADL tasks and reviews targeted task-specific exercises. The OT also helps her purchase a large print pill box, an easy-lock front door, a raised toilet seat so she will not avoid her diuretics due to pain, and a larger scale for the first floor. The RN reviews her medications, suggests lower-sodium frozen vegetable entrees, and brainstorms with Ms. D an action plan to take her medications correctly after identifying that Ms. D is highly motivated to avoid another hospitalization. Your follow-up visit with Ms. D 6 weeks later finds her with a brighter affect, increased adherence to her medical regimen, notable improvement in her symptoms, and overall enhanced functional performance within her home.

Clinical Pearls and Pitfalls

- Performance difficulties with basic ADL and IADL activities in the home result in higher rates of hospital readmissions and overall healthcare costs.
- The home environment, if modified to fit the person, enhances adherence with medical recommendations/plan of care, promotes safety, provides healthcare savings, and increases a patient's level of independence with ADLs and IADLs.
- Older adults living with chronic conditions, such as heart failure, are at higher risk for cognitive impairment, depression, and visual loss changes resulting in reduced safety

levels affecting functional performance within their home environment.

- A multidisciplinary approach that focuses on assessing a person's health status, home environment, and ability to meet the functional demands within the home results in more effective and efficient methods of delivery for home-based primary care practices.
- Small environmental changes can make big differences.

References

1. Centers for Disease Control and Prevention. The state of vision, aging, and public health in America [Internet]. Atlanta: U.S. Department of Health and Human Services; 2011. Available from: https://www.cdc.gov/visionhealth/pdf/vision_brief.pdf. Accessed 11 Apr 2019.
2. Foster ER, Cunnane KB, Edwards DF, et al. Executive dysfunction and depressive symptoms associated with reduced participation of people with severe congestive heart failure. Am J Occup Ther. 2011;65(3):306–13.
3. Szanton SL, Roth J, Nkimbeng M, et al. Improving unsafe environments to support aging independence with limited resources. Nurs Clin N Am. 2014;49:133–45.
4. Szanton SL, Leff B, Wolff JL, et al. Home-based care program reduces disability and promotes aging in place. Health Aff. 2016;35(9):1558–63.
5. Horowitz BP, Almonte T, Vasil A. Use of the Home Safety Self-Assessment Tool (HSSAT) within community health education to improve home safety. Occup Ther Heal Care. 2016;30(4):356–72.
6. Liu C, Chang W-P, Chang MC. Occupational therapy interventions to improve activities of daily living for community-dwelling older adults: a systematic review. Am J Occup Ther. 2018;72(4):7204190060p1.
7. Szanton SL, Alfonso YN, Leff B, et al. Medicaid cost savings of a preventive home visit program for disabled older adults. J Am Geriatr Soc. 2018;66(3):614–20.
8. Gitlin LN, Winter L, Dennis MP, et al. A randomized trial of a multicomponent home intervention to reduce functional difficulties in older adults. J Am Geriatr Soc. 2006;54(4):809–16.

Chapter 10
Transitioning to Long-Term Care

Namirah Jamshed

Case Study

You take care of Ms. E, a 92-year-old woman with Alzheimer's disease, who lives at home with her daughter. At your first visit 2 years ago, she was independent with all her basic activities of daily living (ADLs). She needed assistance with most instrumental activities of daily living (IADLs). She took no medications at that time. Around that time, her daughter developed breast cancer and began chemotherapy and radiation treatments. Six months ago, you saw Ms. E for a routine visit and noticed some cognitive decline. Her daughter confirmed that Ms. E was then requiring assistance with bathing and dressing, and her daughter was struggling with her own medical problems. At that visit you provided her daughter with a list of resources for taking care of patients with Alzheimer's disease. You also requested for social work to assist her with identifying resources in the community that may be available to her. Now, 6 months later, her daughter calls because Ms. E had a near fall 4 weeks ago while on the way to the bathroom at night. Since that time, she has continued to gradually decline both physically and cognitively. She has lost weight and has a poor appetite. She also appears

N. Jamshed (✉)
UT Southwestern Medical Center, Dallas, TX, USA
e-mail: namirah.jamshed@utsouthwestern.edu

© Springer Nature Switzerland AG 2020
J. L. Colburn et al. (eds.), *Home-Based Medical Care for Older Adults*, https://doi.org/10.1007/978-3-030-23483-6_10

weak. She recognizes her daughter but now needs help with toileting and transfers, and she cannot use the walker without supervision. She can still feed herself.

You make a visit and do a detailed cognitive and functional assessment. She does not appear delirious, and a basic workup is unrevealing for another cause of her gradual functional decline. You conclude that Ms. E's dementia is progressing. Her daughter appears run down during the visit and looks very tired. She has missed two of her own oncology appointments due to challenges with finding someone to watch her mother. She tells you that she feels overwhelmed with her own health issues and doesn't feel she can care for her mother anymore on her own now that Ms. E requires additional help with her ADLs. Her daughter requests assistance with taking care of her mother. You determine that she is suffering from caregiver burden.

My Management

What is your next step in management?

A. Start patient on an acetylcholinesterase inhibitor.
B. Start antipsychotics.
C. Admit to the hospital for evaluation.
D. Refer for home physical and occupational therapy.
E. Assist with transition to assisted living or nursing home.

Diagnosis and Assessment

Alzheimer's dementia is a gradually progressive neurodegenerative disorder. Patients typically gradually decline in cognition and function over 8–10 years. As patients with dementia transition to requiring more assistance with personal care, this is often associated with increased caregiver burden [1]. Patient factors associated with increased likelihood of nursing home placement include dementia (particularly with moderate to advanced dementia, or with behavioral disturbances), dependence in one or more ADLs, and living alone [1–3]. Caregiver factors associated with long-term care placement include high caregiver burden, need for additional assistance with patient care, challenges with the patient's behavioral issues, and caregiver health concerns [3, 4]. Strategies for delaying or preventing long-term care placement depend on individual patient and caregiver characteristics. Studies have shown that occupational therapy and exercise interventions can slow progression of functional decline in dementia, though it is not known if they delay long-term care placement [5]. Educational strategies can help the caregiver to manage behaviors associated with dementia, and employing additional resources (such as paid home health aides) may also help to relieve caregiver burden. Several observational studies have suggested that acetylcholinesterase inhibitors, such as donepezil, may delay placement to a nursing home, though the initial randomized controlled trials did not find this to be true and other trials have shown a time-limited effect [6–8]. Antipsychotics would increase the risk of falls in this patient, and she is not exhibiting behaviors that would warrant consideration of antipsychotics for agitation or safety. Hospital admission is not indicated, as her decline has not been acute, but over several months, there is no evidence of delirium, and workup for reversible causes or infections was unremarkable. Referral for home physical therapy and occupational therapy may help to improve Ms. E's strength and to delay her functional decline, which could help to relieve some of the burden on her daughter if she wanted to try to keep her mother at home [5]. However, given her daughter's expressed need for additional care for her mother and limited financial resources, the preferred option in this scenario is placement in assisted living or long-term care.

Beyond the home setting, long-term care can be provided in assisted living facilities, group homes, or nursing homes (NH), depending on an individual patient's functional status and needs [9]. NH eligibility is determined by state definitions typically based on number and type of ADL impairments. A functional assessment will help to determine the appropriate level of care. For patients with impairment who are directable, adult day centers are an option and can provide respite for the family. These facilities may provide meals, activities, transportation, and hands-on care for those needing assistance with activities of daily living. Some adult day centers specialize in dementia care or mental illness [10]. In assisted living or group home settings, patients require assistance with all IADLs and some ADLs. They may need regular supervision and are unsafe to be left alone or have had a fall recently. They usually require assistance in ambulating or transferring and require assistance with meal preparation but can feed themselves. Patients with dementia who can do their own ADLs with cuing may be able to transition to an assisted living or group home that provides care to patients with dementia, to ensure safety with wandering. Patients who require more assistance (typically with all ADLs) could either remain at the ALF with additional paid caregivers or would transition to nursing home/long-term care. There can be differences in payment structure for assisted living/group home care and nursing home care based on individual states, so it is important to consider options based on state regulations, a patient's insurance coverage (including long term care insurance), and available patient assets. For those with Medicaid, Medicaid waivers may offer additional paid services to individuals who live at home but qualify for a nursing home level of care. This care can be provided at home by a Medicaid-covered personal care assistant or at adult day centers [11]. Figure 10.1 outlines a basic guideline for placement options, based on functional assessment to determine patient care needs.

Management

Once any reversible causes (such as delirium) are ruled out, you focus your attention in assisting the daughter in providing care for her mother. Physical and occupational therapy could assist in strengthening and personal care strategies if

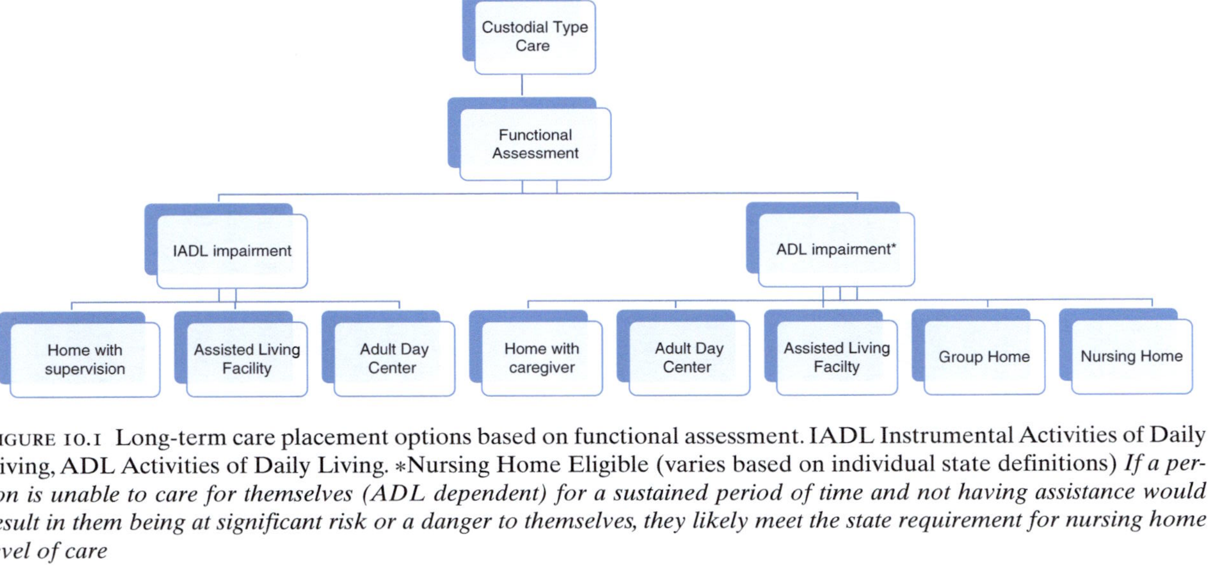

FIGURE 10.1   Long-term care placement options based on functional assessment. IADL Instrumental Activities of Daily Living, ADL Activities of Daily Living. *Nursing Home Eligible (varies based on individual state definitions) *If a person is unable to care for themselves (ADL dependent) for a sustained period of time and not having assistance would result in them being at significant risk or a danger to themselves, they likely meet the state requirement for nursing home level of care*

Ms. E's daughter wants to try to improve her strength and function to see if she can keep her at home. However, home health services (such as PT) would not change her mother's need for 24-hour supervision and would not help with providing supervision and care when Ms. E's daughter must be away from home. Paid home health aides could relieve some of the burden on Ms. E's daughter, though she has limited resources to pay out of pocket and is concerned that they will run out of money quickly for the amount of care that Ms. E will need. In considering medication treatment options, even if medications such as donepezil were to slow the progression of her dementia (questionable based on the evidence), they will not change the need for increased caregiving and personal care assistance at home. In Ms. E's situation, her daughter's caregiver burden is apparent, and she would benefit from respite. In addition, Ms. E has growing care needs with the progression of her dementia, which could be met at home or in a long-term care facility, but her daughter no longer feels she can provide the care.

Outcome

You involve your social worker and plan a family meeting with Ms. E's daughter. You talk with Ms. E's daughter about potential options of additional care at home versus placement in assisted living or nursing home care. Ms. E has some savings that can be used for paid caregiving. However, since she now requires 24/7 supervision and care, those savings will deplete very rapidly. You make a recommendation to the daughter to transition patient to long-term care, to a nursing home setting based on her assets, functional status, and care needs. You ask your social worker to provide ongoing counseling to the daughter for caregiver burden, which she may experience even after her mother is transitioned to long-term care [12]. After a few meetings and with the assistance of the social worker, Ms. E's daughter decides to transition her mother to a nursing home for long-term care.

Clinical Pearls and Pitfalls

(a) As neurodegenerative disorders such as dementia progress, patients exhibit progressive cognitive and functional decline.
(b) Nonpharmacologic interventions, such as exercise programs and physical/occupational therapy, may delay functional decline in patients with dementia.
(c) Caregivers of patients with dementia who require assistance with basic activities of daily living are at higher risk of caregiver burden due to the demands of caregiving.
(d) Medications (including acetylcholinesterase inhibitors) are unlikely to delay cognitive and functional decline associated with dementia.
(e) Antipsychotics should be avoided in older people unless they are needed for safety concerns of patient or caregiver harm resulting from agitation associated with dementia.
(f) Functional status can be used to plan for the need for additional assistance or transition to higher level of care.
(g) Caregiver burden needs to be recognized and may often be the reason for transitioning to placement in long-term care settings.

References

1. Andel R, Hyer K, Slack A. Risk factors for nursing home placement in older adults with and without dementia. J Aging Health. 2007;19(2):213–28.
2. Yaffe K, et al. Patient and caregiver characteristics and nursing home placement in patients with dementia. JAMA. 2002;287(16):2090–7.
3. Gaugler JE, et al. Predictors of nursing home admission for persons with dementia. Med Care. 2009;47(2):191–8.
4. Buhr GT, Kuchibhatla M, Clipp EC. Caregivers' reasons for nursing home placement: clues for improving discussions with families prior to the transition. Gerontologist. 2006;46(1):52–61.

5. McLaren AN, Lamantia MA, Callahan CM. Systematic review of non-pharmacologic interventions to delay functional decline in community-dwelling patients with dementia. Aging Ment Health. 2013;17(6):655–66.
6. Becker M, Andel R, Rohrer L, Banks SM. The effect of cholinesterase inhibitors on risk of nursing home placement among medicaid beneficiaries with dementia. Alzheimer Dis Assoc Disord. 2006;20(3):147–52.
7. Birks JS, Harvey RJ. Donepezil for dementia due to Alzheimer's disease. Cochrane Database Syst Rev. 2018;(6):CD00190.
8. Howard R, McShane R, Lindesay J, et al. Nursing home placement in the Donepezil and Memantine in Moderate to Severe Alzheimer's Disease (DOMINO-AD) trial: secondary and post-hoc analyses. Lancet Neurol. 2015;14(12):1171–81.
9. Residential Facilities, Assisted Living, and Nursing Homes. National Institute on Aging. US Dept of Health & Human Services. https://www.nia.nih.gov/health/residential-facilities-assisted-living-and-nursing-homes. Accessed 11 Apr 2019.
10. Adult Day Centers. Alzheimer's Association. https://www.alz.org/help-support/caregiving/care-options/adult-day-centers. Accessed 30 Apr 2019.
11. Medicaid's Adult Day Care Benefits & Eligibility. American Elder Care Research Association. https://www.payingforseniorcare.com/medicaid-waivers/adult-day-care.html. Accessed 30 Apr 2019.
12. Schulz R, et al. Long-term care placement of dementia patients and caregiver health and well-being. JAMA. 2004;292(8):961–7.

Chapter 11
Pressure Injuries

Yasmin S. Meah, Fred C. Ko, and Elizabeth Arrabito

Case Study

Ms. P is 94 years old and lives at home with her daughter, Elena, who works full time. Ten years ago, Ms. P developed severe osteoarthritis and dementia and was no longer able to care for herself. A paid personal caregiver, Kim, cares for Ms. P during the day. At night, Elena is Ms. P's sole caregiver. Five weeks ago, Ms. P fell while her daughter was transferring her into bed and sustained fractures of the second and third cervical vertebrae. Surgical intervention was not pursued because of the high risk and Ms. P's palliative goals of care. Three days later, Ms. P returned home from the hospital

Y. S. Meah (✉)
Departments of Medicine, Medical Education, Geriatrics and Palliative Medicine, Icahn School of Medicine at Mount Sinai, New York, NY, USA
e-mail: yasmin.meah@mountsinai.org

F. C. Ko
Departments of Geriatrics and Palliative Medicine and Medicine, Icahn School of Medicine at Mount Sinai, New York, NY, USA
e-mail: fred.ko@mssm.edu

E. Arrabito
Departments of Medical Utilization and Care Management, Healthfirst, Inc., New York, NY, USA

© Springer Nature Switzerland AG 2020
J. L. Colburn et al. (eds.), *Home-Based Medical Care for Older Adults*, https://doi.org/10.1007/978-3-030-23483-6_11

with cervical immobilization by rigid collar and skilled home health nursing services.

Four weeks later, the home health nurse calls you. Since returning home, Ms. P has developed multiple pressure injuries of her left and right hips, lower back, and sacrum. The sacrum has the largest pressure injury with an ulcer measuring 10×6 cm with less than 50% viable tissue. The skin around the wound is red and blanches with pressure. The wound margins are not sharp and have a light pink color. There is a moderate amount of exudate and a foul-smelling odor. Her vital signs are normal. The home health nurse has been applying collagenase to the wound daily for chemical debridement, without noticeable improvement. Kim is turning Ms. P every 2 hours during the day. However, at night Ms. P lies supine for up to 8 hours until the late morning when the aide returns. Ms. P is functionally incontinent, and the wound dressings are saturated with urine during the night. Her daughter, Elena, is unable to turn or toilet Ms. P at more frequent intervals due to her full-time work schedule.

My Management

Which of the following interventions should you recommend now?

A. Ensure repositioning of the patient every 6 hours on a static overlay gel mattress (Group 1 support surface).
B. Order antibiotic therapy to treat infection of the sacral ulcer.
C. Begin negative-pressure wound therapy (NPWT).
D. A global assessment of the likelihood of wound healing in the current home environment.

The correct answer is: D

Diagnosis and Assessment

Ms. P was highly vulnerable to pressure-based injury because of her immobility. Pressure injuries often arise in the setting of frailty, acute illness, inadequate repositioning, and poorly mitigated urinary and fecal incontinence. Excessive biofilm, necrosis, and local wound infection delay healing. A global assessment of the likelihood of wound healing in the patients' current home environment is essential. Discussions between patients, caregivers, home care providers, nurses, and social workers should establish a shared understanding of risk factors unique to each patient and realistic goals of wound healing and pain control.

The recommended interval for repositioning patients at high risk for pressure induced injury or those with existing injuries is 2 hours on a standard mattress, up to 4 hours on a pressure-reducing support surface, and every 15 minutes while seated [1]. The evidence behind repositioning intervals is controversial; however, frequent repositioning is an integral part of pressure ulcer prevention and has clear physiologic rationale.

It may be challenging to differentiate infection from normal wound bed bacterial colonization. Reducing bacterial burden in the wound bed requires regular cleansing and irrigation, removing devitalized tissue, appropriate use of antimicrobial dressings, and creating an acidic wound environment that inhibits bacterial proliferation. Signs of infection include fever, spreading erythema around the wound, and increased pain; in such cases, systemic antibiotics are necessary. Negative-pressure wound therapy (NPWT) may be used to accelerate wound healing but is contraindicated for use in pressure injuries with substantial necrotic tissue or eschar [2].

Management

A comprehensive assessment of the likelihood of healing the extensive pressure injuries includes consideration of the following:

1. The overall health of the patient and treatment of underlying conditions
2. Size, stage, and characteristics of the pressure injury
3. Access to necessary durable medical equipment
   Availability of caregivers, both paid of the following:

4. Availability of caregivers, both paid and informal, to ensure scheduled repositioning, handle dressing changes, report concerning changes in wound bed characteristics and control incontinence-induced wetness.

In considering the likelihood of healing, the underlying conditions that led to the pressure injury must be assessed for reversibility. Often underlying frailty, poor nutritional status, severe anemia and compromised circulation due to veno-occlusive disease or congestive heart failure cannot be alleviated. Immobility may not be readily reversible; in such cases, pressure offloading must be implemented to maximize chances of wound healing.

Pressure-reducing and pressure-relieving support surfaces are integral to the care plan [3]. Although data are conflicting, there is consensus that higher-specification foam mattresses as well as air, gel, and water-based surfaces are superior to a standard mattress. Pressure redistribution surfaces are classified as static or dynamic depending on whether they vary the pressure beneath the patient at timed intervals. The Centers for Medicare and Medicaid Services (CMS) has further stratified bed surfaces into three groups based on their degree of pressure reduction or redistribution (see Table 11.1).

Characteristics of the wound itself are also important prognostic factors; these include the wound size and depth, presence of inflammation and bacterial colonization, and vitality of the wound bed. Wound bed preparation to maximize the chances of healing is guided using the TIME (tissue, inflammation/infection, moisture, edge/epithelialization) framework [4, 5]. The general concepts are (1) removal of devitalized and senescent *tissue* through debridement (autolytic, chemical, enzymatic, sharp, and mechanical) to promote the expansion of a healthy extracellular matrix; (2) mitigate and address active *infection and inflammation* by physically removing bacteria and biofilm and choosing appropriate dressings; (3) achieve *moisture* balance through appropriate wound dressings that simultaneously prevent desiccation of the wound bed and reduce excessive moisture to prevent maceration of the

TABLE 11.1 Pressure-relieving support surfaces in home-based medical care

Pressure-relieving surface group	Group 1	Group 2	Group 3
Examples of support surfaces	Gel mattress overlay (static) Alternating pressure pads (dynamic) Static air or gel mattresses	Powered alternating pressure mattress(dynamic) Powered pressure-reducing low-air-loss mattress (dynamic)	Air-fluidized silicone bead beds (dynamic)
Criteria for coverage by Medicare	All persons who are completely immobile OR partially mobile patients and patients with any stage pressure injury with either: Incontinence Poor nutritional state Poor circulation Sensory impairment	Persons must have either multiple stage II pressure injuries on the trunk or pelvis that have not healed or worsened under comprehensive treatment for the past 30 days with the use of a Group 1 support surface OR Large/multiple stage 3 or 4 pressure injuries on the trunk or pelvis OR Recent skin graft or flap for a stage 3 or 4 pressure ulcer	Immobile persons with stage 3 or stage 4 pressure injuries who would require an admission to an inpatient or skilled nursing facility if the device were not provided *and* have previously failed therapy with a Group 2 device

Adapted from *Geriatric Home-Based Medical Care* (p. 219) by JL Hayashi, B Leff B (Eds), 2016, Switzerland: Springer International. Copyright 2016 by Springer International Publishing. Adapted with permission [6]

wound edge; and (4) protect and promote the advancement of the *edge* of the wound bed, and use fillers and dressings that optimize *epithelial* growth.

Outcome

The interdisciplinary care team engaged in detailed discussions with the daughter about the plan of care and how difficult it was to manage the patient in the home based on the above considerations. A skilled home health nurse visited Ms. P several times a week to provide wound bed management to the multiple pressure injuries, but the aide was unable to administer opiates just prior to her visits; as a result, wound management visits took inordinately long and were frequently interrupted or prematurely halted due to poorly controlled pain. Both mechanical and sharp debridement were performed at the bedside. Because the drainage of these ulcers ranged from moderate to severe, the cavities were filled with absorptive dressings. Significant layering with secondary dressings was used to protect against moisture from feces and urine. A dynamic Group 2 low-air-loss mattress was obtained, but the wounds continued to decline. The daughter revealed that despite her best intentions she was unable to turn the patient at an interval more frequent than once every 6 hours overnight and required more hours of home attendant services; this was not granted by the skilled home care agency. The interdisciplinary team met with the family to discuss overall prognosis. Ms. P's goals of care are comfort-focused, and her priority was to remain home. Given the poor prognosis for wound healing, Ms. P was referred to home hospice.

Clinical Pearls and Pitfalls

- Home care providers should be familiar with the indications for use of pressure-reducing support surfaces and consider them part of the armamentarium of home-based wound care.

- The TIME framework helps steer management decisions on local wound management; additionally, the home care provider should consider regional, systemic, and environmental factors as equally critical.
- An interdisciplinary team approach can help ensure that caregiver support is maximized when caring for patients with complex wounds. The home care provider should align goals of care with a realistic assessment of how likely pressure injuries are to heal in the current home environment.

References

1. McInnes E, Dumville JC, Jammali-Blasi A, Bell-Syer SE. Support surfaces for treating pressure ulcers. Cochrane Database Syst Rev. 2011;(12):CD009490.
2. Orgill D, Bayer L. Negative pressure wound therapy: past, present and future. Int Wound J. 2013;10:15–9.
3. Rich SE, Margolis D, Shardell M, et al. Frequent manual repositioning and incidence of pressure ulcers among bedbound elderly hip fracture patients. Wound Repair Regen. 2011;19(1):10–8.
4. Schultz GS, Sibbald RG, Falanga V, et al. Wound bed preparation: a systematic approach to wound management. Wound Repair Regen. 2003;11:S1–S28.
5. Alvarez OM, Kalinski C, Nusbaum J, et al. Incorporating wound healing strategies to improve palliation (symptom management) in patients with chronic wounds. J Pall Med. 2007;10(5):1161–89.
6. Meah YS, Gliatto PM, Ko FC, Skovran D. Wound care in home-based settings. In: Hayashi JL, Leff B, editors. Geriatric home-based medical care: principles and practice. 1st ed. Switzerland: Springer; 2016. p. 195–236.

Chapter 12
Opioid Management

Elizabeth McCormick and Meng Zhang

Case Study

Ms. Q is a 78-year-old woman with osteoporosis and chronic low back pain due to severe degenerative disease. Her gait has become increasingly unsteady, and she has had several falls in the past year. Her last fall was 2 weeks ago. She went to the emergency room, where imaging revealed acute vertebral compression fractures at L3 and L4. She was prescribed tramadol 100 mg three times daily for pain control when discharged from the emergency room. It has not been effective. Since then she has become increasingly homebound and was referred to your home-based medical care practice. She lives in a third-floor walk-up apartment and has a paid caregiver who assists her with personal care for a few hours a day but is otherwise alone. A niece lives nearby and occasionally visits.

On your initial visit, you find Ms. Q alert, engaging, and knowledgeable of her medical problems. She is attentive to self-care and her apartment is clean but cluttered. Her cognition is fully intact. Her major complaint is ongoing back pain. She describes chronic lower back pain for years; however, her

E. McCormick (✉) · M. Zhang
Mount Sinai Visiting Doctors Program, Department of Medicine & Department of Geriatrics and Palliative Medicine, Icahn School of Medicine at Mount Sinai, New York, NY, USA
e-mail: elizabeth.mccormick@mountsinai.org

J. L. Colburn et al. (eds.), *Home-Based Medical Care for Older Adults*, https://doi.org/10.1007/978-3-030-23483-6_12

pain has increased markedly since her most recent fall and compression fractures, and this has significantly impaired her functional abilities. On physical examination, she has severe pain over the L3–L4 region to palpation, as well as paraspinal and tenderness in her lumbar area. Pain worsens substantially with movement. Neurologic examination reveals no focal weakness and intact deep tendon reflexes but is notable for mild decreased tactile sensation in her feet. She has difficulty changing positions due to pain, her gait is unsteady, and she is kyphotic. She is in severe pain with walking.

She also has a history of hypertension, peptic ulcer disease with history of upper gastrointestinal bleed (UGIB), and depression. Her medications are acetaminophen, losartan, chlorthalidone, and pregabalin 50 mg three times daily.

Previously, Ms. Q reports that she had been followed for the past 20 years at a local internal medicine ambulatory practice and reports that her chronic lower back pain was attributed to "arthritis" and has been treated at various times with acetaminophen, nonsteroidal anti-inflammatory drugs (NSAIDs), tramadol, oxycodone, morphine, and lidocaine patches. She has gone to the emergency department multiple times for worsening back pain, particularly over the past 2 years.

She shares that she has been feeling "down" in the last year, and increasingly so over the last few weeks. She has lived in the neighborhood for more than 50 years and was active outside her home but now feels increasingly isolated and "stuck" with her worsening pain and mobility.

My Management

In addition to assessing Ms. Q's physical function and related pain issues and making a diagnosis as to the likely etiology of her back pain, which of the following should you do now?

A. Prescribe gabapentin.
B. Prescribe a short acting higher potency opioid analgesic.
C. Prescribe tramadol at higher dose.

D. Prescribe NSAID.

E. Increase her pregabalin dose.

Answer: B

Diagnosis and Assessment

You complete a comprehensive history, including an assessment of the pain level and characteristics, alleviating and exacerbating factors, and associated symptoms, as well as impact of pain on function and mood [1]. Treating Ms. Q's pain requires a comprehensive approach, ideally with an interdisciplinary team that can provide ongoing primary care in the home. Her pain is severe, and her function has been severely limited by it. The natural history of pain associated with acute vertebral fractures is that of resolution within approximately 3 months. While there is little evidence in literature demonstrating the benefit of long-term opioid use in chronic low back pain, you believe Ms. Q will benefit from short-term opioid use due to the severity of her acute pain from her compression fractures. Her pain is not neuropathic and would likely not respond to gabapentin or augmentation of her pregabalin. She has already failed a robust dose of tramadol, and NSAIDs are to be avoided given her prior UGIB.

Management

The CDC Guidelines for Prescribing Opioids for Chronic Pain [2] can be useful in providing guidance for the management of Ms. Q's pain. These guidelines highlight the importance of setting treatment goals including functional goals, incorporating non-pharmacologic and non-opioid therapy, and discussing with patients the risks and benefits of opioid therapy. Assessment should include screening patients for risk of misuse and a check of state physician drug monitoring portals. When prescribing long-term opioid therapy, the provider should consider use of a pain agreement and periodic drug testing. You also explain to Ms. Q that as her pain and function improve, you will taper her off the opioid [3].

Opioids are not appropriate in every case of acute pain, especially if the risk for misuse is high. Before prescribing opioids, you assess the patient for risk of future misuse of opioids using a tool such as the Opioid Risk Tool [4], a self-report screening tool, which can be completed in about 1 minute. In the absence of personal or family history of alcohol, illegal drug, or prescription drug abuse or serious mental illness, including depression, the risk of misuse is low, as was the case of Ms. Q.

Compared with managing opioid use in patients in ambulatory primary care, there are advantages to managing opioids in the context of home-based medical care. The home provides a real-life setting to assist patients with medication management and assess functional status. Homebound patients may also benefit from Medicare skilled home health services. With the assistance of a home health nurse, the clinician can closely monitor patient's response, side effects, and aberrant behaviors that may be associated with opioid use. Home health nurses can also help educate patient and caregivers, ensure adherence, and assist with correct use. Frequent communication with the home health nurse helps the medical provider initiate, titrate, and taper opioid in a timely manner. In addition, the home health nurse can refer to the home health agency's social worker to help address psychosocial concerns and physical and occupational therapists to help to maximize Ms. Q's function and empower the patient to manage her disease.

Outcome

The next week, the home health nurse calls you with an update on Ms. Q's status. She reports that the patient began taking short-acting oxycodone 5 mg every 8 hours for her pain, which provides excellent pain control. Had she required higher doses of oxycodone, you may have considered using a long-acting regimen of oxycontin with 10% of her total daily dose of short-acting oxycodone for breakthrough [5]. Ms. Q reports improvement in her pain and increased ability to complete some activities of daily living, such as bathing and dressing as well as ability to participate in physical therapy.

Ms. Q is not experiencing any side effects from the oxycodone. With her pain under better control, she has been more social with her neighbors. She is also motivated to work with home physical and occupational therapy. You recognize and empower her by affirming the positive changes she has made. Ms. Q shares that she felt some relief after meeting with the community social worker to whom you referred her. It was helpful to have someone to talk to, and the social worker is also arranging meal delivery and further support at home.

You visit Ms. Q in another few weeks and note her improved functional status and pain control and discuss goal of tapering her off opioids as her acute pain due compression fracture is resolving. You adjust the rate of tapering based on Ms. Q's response and symptoms of withdrawal.

Clinical Pearls and Pitfalls

- When prescribing opioids consider age, comorbidities, type of pain, prior experience with opioids, risk of misuse, and ability to use safely in home.
- Focus on improving or maintaining functional status, empowering patient self-management, and realistic goal setting.
- Incorporate non-pharmacological interventions and non-opioid therapy into the treatment plan.
- Counsel about side effects, prescribe a bowel regimen, and discuss risks of misuse, the importance of safe storage, and the plan to taper opioids used in management of acute pain.

References

1. American Academy of Family Practice. AAFP chronic pain management toolkit. https://www.aafp.org/dam/AAFP/documents/patient_care/pain_management/cpm-toolkit.pdf. Accessed 11 Apr 2019.
2. Centers for Disease Control and Prevention. Guideline for prescribing opioids for chronic pain. Atlanta: U.S. Department of Health and Human Services. https://www.cdc.gov/drugoverdose/pdf/Guidelines_Factsheet-a.pdf. Accessed 11 Apr 2019.
3. Centers for Disease Control and Prevention. Pocket guide: tapering opioids for chronic pain. Atlanta: U.S. Department of Health and Human Services. https://www.cdc.gov/drugoverdose/pdf/clinical_pocket_guide_tapering-a.pdf. Accessed 11 Apr 2019.
4. Webster LR, Webster RM. Predicting aberrant behaviors in opioid-treated patients: preliminary validation of the Opioid Risk Tool. Pain Med. 2005;6(6):432–442. Available for download at https://www.drugabuse.gov/sites/default/files/files/OpioidRiskTool.pdf.
5. Gammaitoni AR, Fine P, Alvarez N, et al. Clinical application of opioid equianalgesic data. Clin J Pain. 2003;19(5):286–97.

Chapter 13
Social Isolation

Thomas K. M. Cudjoe and Jessica L. Colburn

Case Study

Ms. R is a 74-year-old woman recently hospitalized after she experienced a fall with injury at home. She was discharged from the hospital with a referral for home-based physical therapy. The physical therapist referred her to your home-based medical care program, as she has difficulty accessing primary care in the ambulatory setting.

Ms. R has been widowed for 2 years and lives alone in a row home. The row home has two stories, but she lives entirely on the first floor due to mobility challenges associated with osteoarthritis and unsteadiness on her narrow stairs. She ambulates with a front-wheeled walker and has a small half bathroom on the first floor. She spends most of her day on her sofa watching television. She used to crochet but stopped because "there's no point in making things just for myself." She does not smoke, drink alcohol, or use illicit drugs.

She has a past medical history of depression, osteoarthritis, coronary artery disease, and stage III chronic kidney disease. Her medications include metoprolol, lisinopril, aspirin, duloxetine, acetaminophen, vitamin D3, and docusate.

T. K. M. Cudjoe (✉) · J. L. Colburn
Johns Hopkins University School of Medicine, Division of
Geriatric Medicine & Gerontology, Baltimore, MD, USA
e-mail: tcudjoe2@jhmi.edu

© Springer Nature Switzerland AG 2020
J. L. Colburn et al. (eds.), *Home-Based Medical Care for Older Adults*, https://doi.org/10.1007/978-3-030-23483-6_13

You ask her about her social support network, and Ms. R says she has been mostly on her own since her husband, who suffered with dementia, died 2 years ago. She is not involved in any social groups and does not know most of her neighbors because "so many new people are moving in." She used to attend church every Sunday but has not been to church in 10 years, explaining that she stopped going when her husband's dementia progressed and that she has not been able to return since he died. Ms. R previously enjoyed attending book clubs, going to the movie theater with friends, and playing bingo. She says that all the friends she used to have are caring for ill spouses, so she doesn't see them anymore.

An account manager from a nearby neighborhood bank, who has known Ms. R for many years as a regular customer, comes to the house monthly to assist with her bills, and a neighbor helps with shopping for groceries, picking up medications, and other errands. Ms. R has two children but has a strained relationship with them and cannot rely on them for help.

During your house calls, Ms. J is tearful at times, saying that other than her neighbor, "no one would notice if I disappeared." She says she feels lonely but doesn't think she is depressed. She has a good appetite, sleeps well, and does not report suicidal ideation, saying "I could never do that because of my faith."

In exploring her life goals, sense of purpose, and preference for social connections, she says that her faith and connection to religious community is important to her. She also shares that she enjoys people and would like to reconnect but does not feel comfortable leaving her home. She currently does not feel like her life has much purpose.

My Management

Which of the following should you do now?

A. Adjust her antidepressant medications to improve her sadness and isolation.
B. Explore options to increase her social connections, supporting her in connecting with friends, neighbors, and/or church members.

C. Encourage her to start going to clinic instead of being followed by the home-based medical care practice so that she gets out more and sees other people.
D. Inquire about her relationship with her children.

Diagnosis and Assessment

Social isolation impacts up to one in four older adults [1] and is shown to be an independent risk factor for mortality [2], cognitive decline [3], and hospitalization due to heart failure [4]. Social isolation poses a unique risk for the health and well-being of homebound older adults.

Is Ms. R socially isolated? The Lubben Social Network Scale [5] (see Table 13.1) assesses risk of isolation based on contact with relatives and friends seen over the course of a month, how many they feel they can talk to about private matters, and how many they feel close enough to call on for help.

TABLE 13.1 Lubben Social Network Scale-6 (LSNS-6)

FAMILY: Considering the people to whom you are related by birth, marriage, adoption, etc.	0 = none 1 = one
1. How many relatives do you see or hear from at least once a month?	2 = two 3 = three or four
2. How many relatives do you feel at ease with that you can talk about private matters?	4 = five thru eight
3. How many relatives do you feel close to such that you could call on them for help?	5 = nine or more
FRIENDSHIPS: Considering all of your friends including those who live in your neighborhood	0 = none 1 = one
4. How many of your friends do you see or hear from at least once a month?	2 = two 3 = three or four
5. How many friends do you feel at ease with that you can talk about private matters?	4 = five thru eight
6. How many friends do you feel close to such that you could call on them for help?	5 = nine or more

Scores on the LSNS 6 range from 0 to 30; higher scores indicate more social connection. A score less than 12 is considered at risk for social isolation, for instance, if an individual has only one relative and one friend that they see over the course of a month, feel they can talk to about private matters, and feel close enough to call on for help. Based on the LSNS 6, they are at risk for social isolation. This is also true for Ms. R who scores a six on the LSNS 6.

A variety of factors contribute to Ms. R's social isolation, including estrangement from her children, isolation from other friends and social interactions resulting from caring for a spouse with dementia, and her homebound status.

Management

You express your concern to Ms. R that her social isolation is contributing to her sense of loneliness and could lead to additional negative health outcomes, and she states that she would like to consider options to connect with others and is agreeable to coming up with an action plan. To further explore available community resources and support, you connect Ms. R with the social worker from the home health agency to assist her with identifying other options.

After working with her physical therapist, she identifies that leaving the home is a barrier to her social connections. She is not able to afford to install a ramp and is not comfortable exploring solutions that involve leaving her home. She sets a goal of reaching out to her former church to see if someone would visit her weekly to bring communion and pray with her. She also is agreeable to talking and working with the social worker on repairing relationships with her children.

You consider whether to adjust her antidepressants, but she does not endorse symptoms of depression other than feeling lonely and that her life lacks purpose. She brightens when talking about ways she might improve connections with others and prefers not to change her antidepressant medications at this time.

Outcome

Ms. R is crocheting when you arrive for your next visit. The social worker visited her several times and helped Ms. R identify some ways to repair her relationships with her children. She says her conversation with her daughter was not easy but that her daughter is open to coming for a visit, which makes Ms. R feel hopeful. She expresses disappointment that her son has not returned her call. Ms. R also spoke with the social worker about activities that she used to enjoy and offered opportunities for connection, including crocheting baby blankets for the local hospital. That discussion led Ms. R to reach out to the local hospital, which does accept homemade baby blankets, and her neighbor agreed to drop them off once a month. This new activity offers her a sense of purpose and enables her to spend the day doing something that she enjoys.

Ms. R has had weekly visits from a member of her church, which she really enjoys. The church volunteer suggested that Ms. R might be interested in hosting a Bible study, book club, or movie discussion in her home for a few church members, which she is considering.

Though she still feels like she spends more time alone than she would like and is disappointed that her son did not return her call, Ms. R now feels more socially connected. She says she is feeling hopeful about her future even though she is not able to leave her home.

Clinical Pearls and Pitfalls

- Absence of social connection has a negative impact on quality of life, medical care, morbidity, and mortality.
- For patients who are homebound, social history taking should include a discussion about social connection preferences, existing social supports and connections, sense of purpose, and community resources.
- Screening for depression and anxiety as well as conducting a functional status assessment are important pieces of

understanding potential barriers to social connections in homebound older adults.
- Relatives, friends, and neighbors can be an important resource for socially isolated older adults.
- Community resources such as senior centers, religious groups, and social clubs can be a source of beneficial social connection for homebound seniors.
- Social workers and case managers can offer information about existing services and community resources that might support homebound seniors at risk or experiencing social isolation.

References

1. Cudjoe TKM, Roth DL, Szanton SL, et al. The epidemiology of social isolation: National Health & Aging Trends Study. J Gerontol B Psychol Sci Soc Sci. 2018; https://doi.org/10.1093/geronb/gby037. [Epub ahead of print]
2. Holt-Lundstad J, Smith TB, Layton JB. Social relationships and mortality risk: a meta-analytic review. PLoS Med. 2010;7(7):e10000316.
3. Wilson RS, Krueger KR, Arnold SE, et al. Loneliness and risk of Alzheimer disease. Arch Gen Psychiatry. 2007;64(2):234–40.
4. Cene CW, Loehr L, Lin FC, et al. Social isolation, vital exhaustion, and incident heart failure: findings from the Atherosclerosis Risk in Communities Study. Eur J Heart Fail. 2012;14(7):748–53.
5. Lubben J, Blozik K, Gillmann G, et al. Performance of an abbreviated version of the Lubben Social Network Scale among three European community-dwelling older adult populations. Gerontologist. 2006;46(4):503–13.

Chapter 14
Serious Mental Illness

Sonica Bhatia and M. Victoria M. Kopke

Case Study

Robert, the only son of your 87-year-old patient Ms. S, calls you on Monday morning and says "Mom hasn't been doing well and is saying strange things."

Ms. S has hypertension, chronic obstructive pulmonary disease (COPD), obesity, bilateral knee osteoarthritis, and a history of depression. She walks with a two-wheeled rolling walker and is homebound due to pain with walking from her osteoarthritis and dyspnea from her COPD. She was referred to your home-based primary care practice because of difficulty accessing office-based care.

She was diagnosed with depression many years ago following her husband's death. She has been taking sertraline 50 mg daily for over 10 years. In addition to her antidepressant, her current medications include lisinopril, as-needed acetaminophen, tiotropium, and an as-needed albuterol inhaler.

Ms. S lives alone in her apartment. A cleaning person comes weekly, and Robert comes by monthly to help with paying the bills and has set up a weekly grocery delivery service. When you saw her last month for a routine house call,

S. Bhatia (⊠) · M. V. M. Kopke
The Mount Sinai Health System, New York, NY, USA
e-mail: sonica.bhatia@mountsinai.org;
victoria.kopke@mountsinai.org

© Springer Nature Switzerland AG 2020
J. L. Colburn et al. (eds.), *Home-Based Medical Care for Older Adults*, https://doi.org/10.1007/978-3-030-23483-6_14

Ms. S scored a 23/30 on the Montreal Cognitive Assessment (MoCA).

Robert notes that 1 month ago, his mother's friend had mentioned that Ms. S has not been joining her at their twice-weekly chair exercise class, which is unusual for her. This past Friday, when Robert called his mother, she said that the neighbors are spying on her and the people in the pictures on her wall were also watching her and laughing. Robert calls you regarding these symptoms.

You visit Ms. S the following day. You know that Ms. S prides herself on her appearance and neat home. However, at this visit, the apartment is dark as she has all the blinds closed. Her clothes are stained and dirty; her sink is filled with unwashed dishes. You see a stack of unread newspapers in the living room. In her refrigerator you find new groceries but that she hasn't removed the old containers of spoiled milk. There are empty medication bottles on her dining room table. On the kitchen counter, you find a bag from the pharmacy dated 2 weeks ago with unopened pill bottles inside.

Sitting down to speak with Ms. S., she becomes tearful, saying she is upset that her neighbors have been watching her. She says she knows the apartment isn't as clean-looking as she likes it, but she just hasn't had the energy. When asked if she is having any thoughts of harming herself or others, she says "Heavens no, only the Good Lord gets to decide when we leave this planet." She scores a 10 on the 15-question Geriatric Depression Scale (GDS), indicating moderate depression. She has no other physical symptoms or complaints.

On exam, she is alert and her gait is symmetric using her rolling walker. Her blood pressure is 158/72 mmHg, heart rate 77 per minute, and temperature 98.2° Fahrenheit. Her physical examination, including a neurological examination, is otherwise unremarkable. She is awake, alert, fully attentive, and oriented to herself and her address but cannot name the year or month.

You draw a complete blood count, comprehensive metabolic panel, and thyroid stimulating hormone level, which are all within normal limits.

My Management

Which of the following is the most appropriate next step?

A. Return home visit to re-evaluate Ms. S later in the week after her son returns home.
B. Discontinue lisinopril as she may be experiencing an acute adverse reaction.
C. Prescribe olanzapine 2.5 mg daily for depression with psychotic features and refer to skilled home nursing for medication monitoring.
D. Call 911 to bring her to the emergency department of the local hospital for emergency psychiatric evaluation.
E. Increase sertraline from 50 to 100 mg daily to treat depression.

Answer: C

Diagnosis and Assessment

Ms. S's acute symptoms of psychosis and moderate depression are most consistent with a diagnosis of depression with psychotic features.

The differential diagnosis of acute changes in behavior and thought process include delirium, adverse medication reaction, advancing dementia, late-onset schizophrenia, and mood disorders [1]. Infections and electrolyte disturbances can contribute to delirium, but while her thinking has paranoid features and is disorganized, she is fully attentive and alert, without signs of fluctuations in her level of attentiveness or consciousness.

Seeing Ms. S at home enables the physician to see all the pill bottles, including OTC medications and supplements, and ask the patient about them. It is critical to review all medications, as many commonly used medications such as anticholinergic medications including diphenhydramine (which is present in many OTC sleep aids), nonsteroidal anti-inflammatory drugs (NSAIDs), dopaminergic agents, and even dextromethorphan found in cough medications can cause a change in mental status. Lisinopril, however, is unlikely to be the culprit in this case.

Late-onset schizophrenia is characterized by delusions, hallucinations, bizarre behavior, and thought disorder. While Mrs. S. exhibits some symptoms that are consistent with late-onset schizophrenia, this is unlikely the case because of the rapidity of the development of symptoms, her prior history of depression, lack of prior history of psychosis, and lack of bizarre and complex delusions.

Approximately 1–5% of older adults suffer from major depression at any given time [2], and over 14% of depressed individuals have a psychotic episode [3]. The elderly are more likely to have a psychotic episode accompany their depression compared with younger cohorts [4]. Depression in older adults is under-recognized and undertreated, perhaps because of its atypical presentation [2, 5]. Younger people with depression most often present with mood symptoms, while older adults tend to present with somatic complaints, anhedonia, and cognitive impairment [2]. Furthermore, patients with depression may not be able to make it to a doctor's office because of their level of apathy or cognitive impairment. Seeing a patient's home environment may reveal dysfunction that was not apparent during an office visit such as evidence of self-neglect or of substance abuse.

Depression with psychotic features is more severe than depression without psychotic features and often results in increased incapacity for a longer time with an increased likelihood of recurrence [3]. Patients with mood disorders with psychosis show greater cognitive decline than those whose mood disorders are without accompanying psychosis [4] and co-occurring anxiety is common [3].

Management

First-line treatment for depression with psychotic features should include an antidepressant and antipsychotic given concomitantly or electroconvulsive therapy (ECT) [4, 6].

Often these medications can be started while keeping the patient in their home. However, if there is not sufficient oversight in the home setting, it is reasonable to request a hospital admission while initiating and titrating these medications. Other reasons to consider emergency department evaluation and admission include suicidality, severe self-neglect, or violent behavior. While there have been few randomized controlled trials at this time, initiating an antidepressant and antipsychotic in tandem seems to produce better outcomes than either type of medication alone [7].

The first choice of antidepressant is generally a selective serotonin reuptake inhibitor (SSRI) rather than a serotonin-norepinephrine reuptake inhibitor (SNRI) or a tricyclic antidepressant (TCA) because SSRIs tend to have fewer side effects [8]. Choice of specific antipsychotic medications is based on expert consensus guidelines, which recommend the use of atypical antipsychotic medications such as risperidone, olanzapine, or quetiapine [1]. Possible side effects of antipsychotics include parkinsonism, tardive dyskinesia, and akathisia, particularly with first-generation antipsychotics. Weight gain, dyslipidemia, and hyperglycemia are common with clozapine and olanzapine [9]. Older adults should be monitored closely for these side effects.

In contrast to depression in younger patients, the general recommendation for treating depression in older adults is to continue pharmacological treatment indefinitely [5]. In addition to drug treatment, we recommend exercise, improving nutrition, and increasing social interactions [8], all of which can be more challenging to accomplish for geriatric homebound populations.

ECT has been found to be as effective a treatment for depression with psychotic features and has the benefit of faster improvement in depressive symptoms [4]. Access to ECT for the homebound population is challenging, as the patient must be able to leave the home to be evaluated by a psychiatrist and also for multiple outpatient ECT sessions and are required to have someone accompany them to all outpatient ECT sessions.

Outcome

After evaluating Ms. S and speaking with her and with her son Robert by phone, you feel secure in keeping her at home and treating her with combination drug therapy. Robert is arriving the next morning and is able to stay with his mother for several weeks. You initiate a skilled home health care episode, so a nurse will help with medication management and education.

You continue sertraline 50 mg daily and add a low-dose second-generation antipsychotic, olanzapine 2.5 mg daily. You suggest that until the patient's status improves, Robert must administer Ms. S's medications. In addition, Robert hires a paid personal caregiver for 4 hours a day 7 days a week to help Ms. S with bathing, dressing, and meal preparation. When you see her again in 2 weeks, she appears less paranoid, and her GDS score is now 7. Her appetite and self-care have improved. Her paranoid ideation has improved. Her mood is still low. You increase her sertraline to 100 mg and continue olanzapine at 2.5 mg daily. You see her again 1 month later, and her GDS score is now 5. She is no longer paranoid and is attending her chair exercise class again. Robert has returned to his home, and Ms. S. is able to administer her own medications with a daily pill box. You plan to evaluate her in another month to see if olanzapine can be stopped and if her paid personal caregiver hours can be reduced.

Clinical Pearls and Pitfalls

- The presentation of new-onset depression in older adults can be atypical and may present with irritability, psychotic symptoms, and cognitive decline rather than prominent mood symptoms.
- Given the severity of depression with psychotic features, older homebound adults with depression with psychotic features should be treated with an SSRI and antipsychotic. ECT remains a treatment option, but the logistics

of such treatment may be difficult for a homebound frail older adult.

- Assess for suicidality. If the patient is actively suicidal, they should be evaluated in an emergency department. If the patient does not agree to such evaluation, call 911 for assistance.
- Monitor and reduce antipsychotics based on symptoms. Older adults with depression, in contrast to younger adults, often require long-term treatment with SSRIs.

References

1. Reinhardt MM, Cohen CI. Late-life psychosis: diagnosis and treatment. Curr Psychiatry Rep. 2015;17(2):1.
2. Fiske A, Wetherell JL, Gatz M. Depression in older adults. Annu Rev Clin Psychol. 2009;5:363–89.
3. Wijkstra J, Lijmer J, Burger H, et al. Pharmacological treatment for psychotic depression. Cochrane Database of Syst Rev. 2015;7:CD004044.
4. Wagner GS, McClintock SM, Rosenquist PB, McCall WV. Major depressive disorder with psychotic features may lead to misdiagnosis of dementia: a case report and review of the literature. J Psychiatr Pract. 2011;17(6):432–8.
5. Birrer RB, Vemuri SP. Depression in later life: a diagnostic and therapeutic challenge. Am Fam Physician. 2004;69:2375–82.
6. Alexopoulos GS, Streim J, Carpenter D, Docherty JP. Expert consensus panel for using antipsychotic drugs in older patients. Using antipsychotic agents in older patients. J Clin Psychiatry. 2004;65(Suppl 2):5–99.
7. Meyers BS, Flint AJ, Rothschild AJ, et al; STOP-PD Group. A double-blind randomized controlled trial of olanzapine plus sertraline vs olanzapine plus placebo for psychotic depression: the study of pharmacotherapy of psychotic depression (STOP-PD). Arch Gen Psychiatry. 2009;66(8):838–47.
8. Solomon CGE, Taylor WD. Depression in the elderly. N Engl J Med. 2014;371:1228–36.
9. Muench J, Hamer AM. Adverse effects of antipsychotics medications. Am Fam Physician. 2010;81(5):617–22.

Chapter 15
Functional Rehabilitation and Realistic Goals

Jennifer Hayashi and Cindy Seidenman

Case Study

Mr. U is an 87-year-old man with dementia, depression, hypertension, diabetes, atrial fibrillation, congestive heart failure, and osteoarthritis. Three months ago, he was living in his own two-story home with minor assistance from his daughter Mary, who visited every morning before work to help him with meal preparation and taking his medications. He was walking independently with a rolling walker at that time.

Unfortunately, he sustained a mechanical fall in his bathroom and was taken to the hospital, where he was observed for 24 hours, and discharged to Mary's home with a plan to transition back to his own home in a few days. In the hospital, Mr. U had negative imaging studies of the hip, pelvis, and head.

While at Mary's home, Mr. U refused to get out of bed for a week due to generalized pain and fear of falling. He developed

J. Hayashi (✉)
MedStar House Call Program, Baltimore, MD, USA
e-mail: Jennifer.L.Hayashi@medstar.net

C. Seidenman
John Hopkins Home Care Group, Lutherville, MD, USA

acute shortness of breath and was readmitted to the hospital with a pulmonary embolism. He was discharged to a skilled nursing facility (SNF) for rehabilitation.

SNF staff were able to transfer him from a sitting to standing position using a two-person assist, and he was able to walk a few steps in the parallel bars with assistance. Because he was neither participating fully in skilled therapy nor making progress in his functional status, he was discharged home with physical and occupational therapy after 12 days in the SNF.

You are the physician seeing Mr. U at home as a new patient. Since returning to Mary's home, he again has not gotten out of bed. His mental status has been normal. Mary wants her father to move in with her permanently. Mr. U wants to go back to his own home. Mary is having difficulty caring for her father and has no help from extended family or community. Mr. U is staying in a bedroom on the second floor because it is close to the bathroom. He has a hospital bed and a bedside commode. Mary asks you and the home physical therapist (PT) and occupational therapist (OT) for help and advice. Current medications include acetaminophen, lisinopril, furosemide, metformin, sertraline, and apixaban.

On examination, Mr. U has normal vital signs without orthostatic changes. He denies significant pain or dyspnea at rest or with activity. He can get to a sitting position on the edge of the bed but cannot stand without you and Mary both helping him.

My Management

Which of the following should you do next?

A. Advise Mary to consider a nursing home for her father.
B. Order a mechanical lift to begin caregiver training.
C. Discuss Mr. U's and Mary's goals of treatment.
D. Send Mr. U to the emergency department to rule out subdural hematoma.

Answer: C

Diagnosis and Assessment

Accurate diagnosis and optimal management require close collaboration among the home-based medical provider, PT, OT, caregiver, and patient. Mary is clearly committed to keeping her father at home, so referring her to local nursing homes could endanger the developing therapeutic relationships between her and the home-based medical care team. A mechanical lift is not appropriate now because he may still progress with therapy to regain the ability to transfer without it. Given unremarkable imaging, some functional improvement in the SNF, and a clear sensorium since his return home, a subdural hematoma, occult fracture, or other medical issue is unlikely to be the cause of his immobility.

Mr. U most likely has an acute functional decline superimposed on chronic debility exacerbated by fear of falling and depression. His comorbidities, including dementia and depression, limit his ability to recover function, follow through on a home exercise program, and live safely by himself. His situation is further complicated by caregiver burden and lack of social support.

The role of the home-based medical care team is to optimize Mr. U's chance for successful home-based recovery of function and to help Mary recognize and accept the limits of such recovery. Understanding and reconciling Mr. U's and Mary's goals is an important first step in fulfilling this role.

Management

The PT and OT will evaluate the patient's physical and cognitive abilities and home environment to formulate an initial plan of care. Patient and caregiver safety, both physical and emotional, is the first consideration in establishing a rehabilitation plan. Minimizing the risk of physical harm may depend on a loss of autonomy that is unacceptable to the patient. Multiple factors (see Table 15.1) influence the therapist's assessment of "rehabilitation potential," or the likelihood

TABLE 15.1 Factors affecting rehabilitation potential

Intrinsic factors	Extrinsic factors
Psychological factors (motivation, spirituality, confidence)	Home setup (see Chaps. 8 and 9, "Falls Management" and "Home Safety Risk Assessment" for details)
Cognition	Neighborhood safety
Medical conditions	Informal support
Polypharmacy	Family/caregiver goals
Abnormal vital signs (e.g., orthostatic hypotension, symptomatic arrhythmias)	Physician involvement
Pain	
Anxiety/depression	
Previous level of function	
Duration of disability	

that the patient will be able to return to their previous level of function [1]. An occupational therapist will focus on the ability to complete activities of daily living (ADLs), and a physical therapist will focus on balance, strength, and mobility.

Establishing realistic functional goals requires consideration of each of these multiple variables, specific to each patient's situation. Mr. U was living alone and ambulating independently with a rolling walker only 3 months ago. He appears motivated to return to independent living, but his depression, dementia, and fear of falling will impact his progress. Mary is also motivated for her father to become independent, but her goals for his living situation differ from his. The home care therapists can incorporate features of his home environment, such as furniture, appropriate durable medical equipment (DME), and the physical layout of each room, into a plan of care that will optimize his ability to perform his ADLs.

Mr. U's multiple comorbidities increase the likelihood that he will continue to require some assistance in the short term. As he ages, he will probably require more assistance over time. Discussions balancing his desire for autonomy with his physical safety, risk of falls, and need for supervision should occur over multiple visits and be addressed by each team member. As home therapy continues, the PT and OT will provide ongoing reassessment of reasonable goals based on his cognition and his physical abilities and may break goals down into smaller objectives to help him maintain his motivation and progress.

Communication among the PT, OT, physician, Mr. U, and Mary is crucial to optimizing Mr. U's functional recovery. Each health care discipline has distinct areas of expertise, and collaboration between these areas is more likely to lead to creative problem-solving [2]. Each can also build rapport with Mary and Mr. U over time as they work to improve his trajectory of illness and functional impairment. This rapport may help the clinicians have frank discussions about prognosis if Mr. U is unable to return to his prior level of function. Importantly, the PT, OT, and physician should agree if and when those discussions should occur, to prevent confusion or conflicting expectations.

Outcome

You and the therapists agree that the ideal situation would be to have Mr. U move in with Mary permanently, to both decrease Mary's caregiver burden and allow Mr. U some independence during the day. At first Mr. U disagrees with the recommendation but reluctantly agrees to a trial period in Mary's home. Over the next few weeks, he makes slow, steady progress with therapy. He is able to walk with the rolling walker short distances independently but still requires assistance on steps and with bathing. Mr. U begins to realize, with the guidance of the team whom he has grown to trust, that he does need Mary's help. He agrees that returning to his home is not feasible due to his home setup and lack of needed assistance and decides to stay with Mary permanently. Mr. U's mood and his fear of falling improve as he gains confidence in his abilities. The PT recommends referral to the skilled home health agency's social worker for identification of community support services and long-term planning.

Clinical Pearls and Pitfalls

- Patient and caregiver safety should always be balanced with autonomy and function in establishing a rehabilitation plan.
- Realistic goal setting requires consideration of multiple issues, specific to patient circumstances. Knowledge of the home environment can be leveraged to develop an effective plan that achieves the goals of care.
- Optimal outcomes require clear and timely communication among the therapists, physician, patient, and caregiver.

References

1. Burton CR, Home M, Woodward-Nutt K, et al. What is rehabilitation potential? Development of a theoretical model through the accounts of healthcare professionals working in stroke rehabilitation services. Disabil Rehabil. 2015;37:1955–60.
2. Strasser DC, Falconer JF, Stevens AB, et al. Team training and stroke rehabilitation outcomes: a cluster randomized trial. Arch Phys Med Rehabil. 2008;89:10–5.

Chapter 16
Polypharmacy

Melissa Morgan-Gouveia

Case Study

Mr. J is an 84-year-old man referred to your home-based medical care program due to difficulty getting to medical appointments. He has a history of coronary artery disease, congestive heart failure, type 2 diabetes, anxiety, and osteoarthritis of the knees.

He has had several recent falls resulting in emergency department visits. Although he has not sustained significant injuries from his falls, he is having more difficulty walking and is now using his walker all the time. Mr. J's main complaints are of substantial fatigue and intermittent dizziness, especially upon standing. During his most recent emergency department visit, his laboratory testing was notable for a BUN of 30 mg/dl and creatinine of 1.3 ml/dl, for which he received intravenous fluids. His hemoglobin was 12 g/dl, and his hemoglobin A1c was 6.2%.

M. Morgan-Gouveia (✉)
Department of Medicine, Christiana Care Health System, Newark, DE, USA

Division of Geriatrics and Gerontology, Johns Hopkins University School of Medicine, Baltimore, MD, USA
e-mail: MMorgan-Gouveia@ChristianaCare.org

© Springer Nature Switzerland AG 2020
J. L. Colburn et al. (eds.), *Home-Based Medical Care for Older Adults*, https://doi.org/10.1007/978-3-030-23483-6_16

During your initial house call, when you ask what medications he is taking, he hands you a list from the hospital that includes aspirin 81 mg daily, atorvastatin 40 mg daily, furosemide 40 mg daily, glyburide 5 mg daily, lisinopril 20 mg daily, lorazepam 0.5 mg daily at bedtime, metformin 1000 mg twice a day, metoprolol succinate 100 mg daily, and paroxetine 20 mg daily.

When you ask to look at his medications, he reluctantly points you to a large grocery store bag filled with over 25 medication bottles. All the medications on his list are present, but there are several duplicate bottles, and a few are old and past expiration. He admits that he sometimes forgets to take his medications or will skip them if he is not feeling well and that he doesn't have a great method to organize his medications. In addition, there are old bottles of isosorbide mononitrate and hydralazine, which he states he is no longer taking. On the table next to his recliner, there are also several over-the-counter medications including ibuprofen and diphenhydramine, which he takes as needed for arthritis pain and itching, respectively.

On exam, Mr. J looks well. His blood pressure is 110/62 mm Hg and heart rate is 48 per minute. When he stands, his blood pressure drops to 88/56 mm Hg, his heart rate increases to 66 per minute, and he feels dizzy. Heart sounds are regular, and his lungs are clear. The skin on his legs is wrinkled, with no edema, and his mouth is dry.

My Management

Which of the following is the most appropriate next step in the management of Mr. J?

A. Prescribe meclizine for dizziness.
B. Refer him to the emergency department for IV fluids.
C. Prescribe fludrocortisone for orthostatic hypotension.
D. Initiate a medication deprescribing process.

Diagnosis and Assessment

Polypharmacy is common among homebound older adults and associated with poor health outcomes including adverse drug events, drug-drug interactions, drug-disease interactions, increased healthcare costs, medication nonadherence, functional impairment, delirium, and falls. Polypharmacy often results from prescribing cascades, where an adverse effect of one medication is treated with another medication. When a patient presents with a new symptom or concern, consider whether the symptom could be a side effect of a medication.

Mr. J is on several medications that can contribute to fatigue, dizziness, and orthostatic hypotension, which may be compounded by taking duplicate or discontinued medications by mistake due to poor organization of his medications. Therefore, it is important to evaluate whether any of these medications can be discontinued before considering prescribing an additional medication to treat his orthostatic hypotension, such as fludrocortisone. It is also important to assist him with organizing his medications and disposing of discontinued and expired medications to reduce the risk of medication errors.

Similarly, it is not appropriate to treat his dizziness with meclizine as this would not address the underlying cause of dizziness and could generate additional adverse effects. Meclizine is highly anticholinergic and would add to his anticholinergic burden in combination with paroxetine and diphenhydramine. While IV fluids may result in short-term symptomatic improvement, they will not address the underlying polypharmacy and therefore not reduce the likelihood of his symptoms recurring. His medication regimen is complex and requires modification through a deprescribing process.

Management

Home-based medical care providers are in an excellent position to obtain an accurate list of the medications a patient is taking by performing medication reconciliation "at the kitchen table." Reviewing pill bottles in the home allows for a complete assessment of medications, including over-the-counter medications that may not be on a patient's medication list but have the potential to interact with their prescription medications or exacerbate their medical conditions. House calls allow providers to observe how patients organize and take their medications and identify barriers to adherence. It is not uncommon for patients to hoard old medications, often due to concerns that they may need them again; this can present safety risks if a patient decides to self-medicate or accidentally takes a medication that has been discontinued. Home-based medical care providers can assist with medication organization and disposal of discontinued or expired medications, reducing the risk of medication errors.

Careful medication review can identify potentially inappropriate medications, and providers can initiate a deprescribing process when the risks outweigh the benefits [1]. Prioritize medications that are high risk in older adults and ones that the patient is willing to discontinue, with the goal of reducing drug-related adverse events and improving function. The Beers Criteria is one available tool to identify potentially inappropriate medications in older adults [2]. It is generally best practice to wean or stop one medication at a time to monitor for withdrawal symptoms or disease rebound. Deprescribing is a collaborative process that involves shared decision-making with patients and consideration of an individual patient's values and preferences, comorbidities, functional status, and life expectancy [1].

Outcome

In Mr. J's case, you discontinued his furosemide and referred him for skilled home nursing and physical therapy. The home health nurse helped him set up a medication planner to organize his medications and informed him how to properly dispose of his old, expired medications. Mr. J found it easier to take his medications out of the pill box, and keeping the pill box on the kitchen table helped him to remember to take his medications daily with his breakfast.

With the nurse's assistance in monitoring vital signs and providing Mr. J with continual education regarding his medications, you were also able, over time, to reduce the dose of his metoprolol and discontinue his glyburide. Further, you switched sertraline for paroxetine, given the substantial anticholinergic effects of the latter. Mr. J's orthostatic hypotension and fatigue both improved. You educated him that non-steroidal anti-inflammatory medications can contribute to fluid retention in heart failure and switched to acetaminophen for his arthritis pain. He also discontinued diphenhydramine after you educated him on the anticholinergic side effects, noting that he doesn't have as much itching now that he is no longer dehydrated and using a moisturizer on his skin like you recommended. His knee pain and walking improved with physical therapy, and he has not had any new falls. He is so pleased with how he is feeling after your deprescribing that he is willing to engage in your other recommendation to attempt to gradually wean off his benzodiazepine.

Clinical Pearls and Pitfalls

- Polypharmacy is common among homebound older adults with multiple chronic conditions and is associated with poor health outcomes.
- Routine home-based medication review and reconciliation are important to identify potentially inappropriate medications, including over-the-counter medications, and to assess medication adherence. The ability to see the actual medications in the patient's home—how they are set up, stored, and organized—can be critical in helping patients with their medication management and adherence.
- Avoid the prescribing cascade, where an adverse effect of one medication is treated with another medication, and always consider non-pharmacologic treatment options before starting a new medication.

- Deprescribing involves shared decision-making with patients and consideration of the potential benefits and harms of a medication in the context of an individual patient's values and preferences, comorbidities, functional status, and life expectancy. Sequential discontinuation of medications with careful observation is advised.

References

1. Scott IA, Hilmer SN, Reeve E, et al. Reducing inappropriate polypharmacy: the process of deprescribing. JAMA Intern Med. 2015;175:827–34.
2. American Geriatrics Society 2019 Beers Criteria update expert panel. American Geriatrics Society 2019 updated AGS beers criteria for potentially inappropriate medication use in older adults. J Am Geriatr Soc. 2019;67:674–94.

Chapter 17
Telephone Medicine

Christian Escobar and Cameron R. Hernandez

Case study

You are the on-call provider for your home-based medical care practice for the weekend. You receive a call in the middle of the night Sunday from Ms. W, an 80-year-old woman with hypertension, osteoarthritis of her hips and knees (which severely limits her ability to leave her home), multiple myeloma, and untreated anxiety. The original text message from your answering service reads: "patient saying she has chest pain and refused 911, wants to speak with a doctor." You scan Ms. W's electronic medical record to find her code status and next of kin. You call, and the patient's husband answers the phone. He says Ms. W has been complaining of belly pain for 2 days and had some vomiting this evening. He gives her the phone, and you speak directly with Ms. W. She reports that she has been having intermittent, diffuse abdominal pain, is achy all over, and the pain is not radiating to her back. She felt burning in her chest after vomiting her dinner earlier in the evening. She says she mentioned chest pain to the operator but clarifies that the pains

C. Escobar (✉) · C. R. Hernandez
Department of Medicine, Department of Geriatrics and Palliative Medicine, Icahn School of Medicine at Mount Sinai,
New York, NY, USA
e-mail: christian.escobar@mountsinai.org

© Springer Nature Switzerland AG 2020
J. L. Colburn et al. (eds.), *Home-Based Medical Care for Older Adults*, https://doi.org/10.1007/978-3-030-23483-6_17

starts in her abdomen. Her medications include hydrochlorothiazide, aspirin, acetaminophen, as well as lenalidomide and dexamethasone prescribed by her oncologist.

My Management

Which of the following should you do next?

A. Send Ms. W to the emergency department via 911 because of initial report of "chest pain" and because abdominal symptoms can be atypical presentation of acute coronary syndrome in older adults.
B. Recommend to Ms. W that she take an antacid and that you will call her back in the morning to assess her status.
C. Tell Ms. W she will receive a visit on the next business day but that you cannot give her medical advice without seeing her in person.
D. Ask follow-up questions about the pain, her prior medical history, and her ability to keep down food and fluids.

Answer: D

Diagnosis and Assessment

Your initial task is to properly triage Ms. W to decide if she needs to go to the emergency department (ED) or if she can wait to see a clinician in the morning. Triaging home-based medical care patients over the telephone, particularly as this population commonly has multiple chronic conditions, functional impairment, and atypical presentation of disease, can be among the most challenging decisions that home-based medical care providers face. Home-based medical care providers often have the advantage of a deep knowledge of the patient's social history and the resources available in their living environment. A chief complaint alone is rarely enough information to make a good triage decision. Asking the patient and caregiver follow-up questions to understand more fully the nature and urgency of the symptoms will help with decision-making.

Management

Reviewing the chart ahead of the call or having it open during the call can aid in decision-making. Urgent calls can be stressful; take a slow, deep breath to mentally prepare for the call. See Table 17.1 for telephone encounter tips.

TABLE 17.1 Tips for an effective and efficient telephone encounter

Tips for an effective and efficient telephone encounter

Review the chart to prepare for the encounter

Introduce yourself clearly with a statement of concern

Use proper clarity and rate of speech

Use a tone of voice that communicates concern and empathy

Verify that you are speaking with the patient or appropriate designee

Use open-ended questions

Encourage the patient to elaborate without interrupting them

Clarify unclear descriptions

Focus on the main problem

Repeat back the patient's history

Ask close-ended/specific question to "fill in the blanks" [1]

Obtain an understanding of how the patient's current condition compares with their baseline

Remember to ask about other/underlying concerns

Seek other sources of information

Consider the patient's goals of care

Give clear call back instructions: what alarming signs to look out for and how to call back

In certain cases, call back a patient within a short timeframe, if needed, to confirm that the patient hasn't deteriorated and to provide additional reassurance

You must first triage the call as urgent and requiring immediate face-to-face evaluation or nonurgent. Consider a person's vital signs, mentation, and ability to take fluids and medication by mouth. If you cannot speak directly to the patient, ask caregivers if they feel the patient is at their normal or baseline state or if they generally look sick. Often a caregiver can be helpful in taking the patient's temperature and checking respiratory rate and pulse. Once you have assessed an individual's symptoms and risk factors, develop a differential diagnosis based on the available information. If your patient has a high likelihood for a life-threatening condition, then referral to an ED via the 911 system is warranted. The ED is also useful in cases where there is a high level of diagnostic uncertainty or testing is required that cannot be done at home, such as a CT scan. For nonurgent cases, timely access to a house call is also a factor in decision-making. Some practices may have the capability of evaluating a patient in person after business hours. However, for many practices, the ability to provide a physician house call at the start of the next day may result in quicker evaluation by a physician than an ED visit in the middle of the night, depending on how busy the ED may be.

Make use of all available resources over the phone, including any home device such as a blood pressure monitor, a pulse oximeter, or a glucometer. Increasingly, patients use technology such as wearable heart rate monitors and even home-based electrocardiogram monitors that may provide useful additional information. Pictures sent by patients and caregivers can also be helpful, especially for dermatologic and wound-related issues. Receiving images is contingent on your institution's regulations and access to a HIPAA complaint modality. Video conferencing to visualize the patient in real time greatly increases the amount of information a provider can assess. Some practices may have ancillary services, such as home imaging (x-rays, ultrasound) and home phlebotomy, which can add valuable information. If a patient is currently receiving skilled home health-care services, skilled nursing may be able to conduct an urgent patient assessment and subsequently discuss with the provider. Finally, some practices have the option of community paramedicine services in which a paramedic can assess a patient and report to the provider by phone or video conferencing. Community paramedics may also be able to administer first-line treatments such as antibiotics, diuretics, or intravenous fluids.

It is important to tailor your recommendations and management to a patient's goals of care. Looking for advanced directives or prior conversations regarding emergencies in the medical record will help guide your management. People that have opted for a palliative approach to care may benefit from reassurance or recommendations for symptom management but may also require the ED if symptoms cannot be controlled at home. Whenever possible, give a sign out to the ED physician since many EDs are not prepared for providing palliative care on site. If the patient has not previously made their preferences known, you may need to discuss these preferences with the patient or caregiver by phone before referring them to the ED. The patient's values, current quality of life, and expectations of care and outcome will help with this decision-making.

Outcome

Ms. W has no history of cardiac or vascular disease. After assessment and questioning, you find that the chest pain is isolated to the burning after emesis. Her main symptom is the abdominal pain and one episode of vomiting. After triaging her as nonemergent, you delve further into her abdominal symptoms such as onset, exacerbating factors, and recent bowel habits. You also ask about other systems, such as urinary symptoms, that may be associated with her situation. You should consider atypical coronary disease, as Ms. W is an older female [2, 3]; however, it is less likely in someone with no prior coronary disease. Abdominal obstruction, constipation, peptic ulcer disease, gallstones, and gastroenteritis are also on her differential diagnosis. Ms. W reports no nausea and that she is passing flatus. You ask her to attempt drinking a few sips of water while you wait on the phone. She is able to take a few sips and then proceeds to finish her entire cup. You reassure her that she is safe to remain at home and recommend that she take acetaminophen as well as an over-the-counter bismuth-containing compound or H2 blocker. Ms. W's husband says he can go to the drug store that night. You encourage drinking at least 2 liters of water over the next 24 hours. You send a message to the home-based medicine scheduler to arrange a clinician visit for the next day. You complete the call by giving the proper call back information in case they have questions or concerns in the middle of the night and explain what to look out for that may warrant a follow-up call, such as worsening pain, hematemesis, or melena.

Ms. W took acetaminophen and an oral antacid overnight and was able to go back to sleep. On the follow-up visit the next day, she appeared to be at her baseline, with normal vital signs and physical examination. She noted that talking directly with the on-call physician and receiving advice from someone who was clearly listening to her helped her avoid an ED visit.

Clinical Pearls and Pitfalls

- When possible, providers should briefly review a patient's medical chart before returning phone calls.
- On the phone, a provider should assess symptoms, availability of resources, and goals of care to inform the key triage decision as to whether the patient requires urgent in-person evaluation or not.
- On-call home-based medical care providers must be familiar with resources that are available during off hours that can help with triage and treatment decisions (e.g., home-based x-rays, nursing, community paramedicine, etc.).

References

1. Stevens DL. In: Reisman AB, editor. Telephone medicine: a guide for the practicing physician. Philadelphia: American College of Physicians; 2002.
2. Panju AA, Hemmelgarn BR, Guyatt GH, et al. Is this patient having a myocardial infarction? JAMA. 1998;280:1256–63.
3. Vaccarino V, Parsons L, Every NR, et al. Sex-based differences in early mortality after myocardial infarction. N Engl J Med. 1999;341:217–25.

Chapter 18
Morbid Obesity

Jean Yudin and Bruce Kinosian

Case Study

You make an initial house call to Mr. X, a 70-year-old man referred to your home-based medical care practice because his obesity makes it too difficult for him to leave his home. He has been referred to you following a recent hospitalization requiring an intensive care unit stay for respiratory failure due to cor pulmonale. This is his fifth hospital admission in the last year. He has required external ventilatory support for hypercapnic respiratory failure during his hospitalizations. He has no nocturnal ventilation support in the home, although it was prescribed at his hospital discharge.

Mr. X's past medical history is notable for oxygen-dependent chronic obstructive pulmonary disease, heart failure with preserved ejection fraction, type 2 diabetes (insulin requiring), obesity hypoventilation syndrome, osteoarthritis,

J. Yudin (✉)
Schnable In Home Primary Care Program, Division of Geriatric Medicine, Perelman School of Medicine, University of Pennsylvania, Philadelphia, PA, USA
e-mail: yudin@pennmedicine.upenn.edu

B. Kinosian
Division of Geriatric Medicine, Perelman School of Medicine, University of Pennsylvania, Philadelphia, PA, USA

© Springer Nature Switzerland AG 2020
J. L. Colburn et al. (eds.), *Home-Based Medical Care for Older Adults*, https://doi.org/10.1007/978-3-030-23483-6_18

and gout. Mr. X's medications are aspirin, atorvastatin, furosemide, long-acting insulin, nebulized bronchodilators, and topical pain medication for his arthritis pain. His daughters fill his pillbox.

Mr. X lives alone in a two-story home with steep entry steps. His first floor is set up with a regular hospital bed and commode, walker, and oxygen per nasal cannula. The doorway from his living room to the kitchen is 36 inches wide (bariatric wheelchairs have an overall width of 32 inches). A private-duty home health aide visits him daily to assist him with bathing, dressing, and grooming. He requires a two-person assist to get to a sitting position at the side of his bed.

Mr. X states he eats three small meals a day with few snacks. An inspection of his kitchen reveals canned soups, microwave popcorn, chips, and sodas.

On exam, Mr. X is alert, although he dozes off during the visit. His blood pressure is 138/60 mm Hg, heart rate 70 bpm, and oxygen saturation 92% on 2 liters oxygen by nasal cannula. His weight is unobtainable, but during his most recent hospitalization, he weighed 380 pounds with a body mass index (BMI) at 39 kg/m². His latest fasting blood sugar is 150 mg/dl. His sacral area and buttocks have excoriations and several small bleeding wounds. Mr. X's daughter is present for the visit and notes that her father is incontinent. Respiratory excursion is diminished. His cardiopulmonary examination is unremarkable. The jugular venous pressure cannot be evaluated due to obesity. There is bilateral brawny lower extremity edema to his thighs.

Mr. X's goals include being out of bed, improved functional status, and avoiding additional hospitalizations. He is interested in losing weight.

My Management

Which of the following should you recommend next?

A. Around-the-clock aide care
B. Bariatric equipment

C. Sleep study and nocturnal bi-level positive airway pressure ventilation (BiPAP)
D. Foley catheter for incontinence
E. B and C

Correct Answer: E

Diagnosis and Assessment

Mr. X is morbidly obese. Morbid obesity is conventionally defined as a BMI > 40, or a BMI > 35 with one or more complications of obesity. Complications of obesity include type 2 diabetes mellitus, hypertension, arthritis, gout, congestive heart failure, and respiratory failure. His problems include lack of mobility due to obesity and lack of appropriate medical equipment in his home and respiratory failure due to obesity hypoventilation syndrome.

Morbid obesity is a common reason for inability to leave the home to access medical care. In-home assessment and ongoing access to care provided by home-based medical care providers can be invaluable in identifying environmental factors such as types of food that limit weight management.

Mr. X does not have financial resources for 24-hour care nor does he need constant supervision. Long-term urinary catheters to manage urinary incontinence pose a high risk of urinary tract infections and are not recommended.

Mr. X's obesity-associated immobility can be ameliorated with properly sized and supportive equipment including a bariatric bed for pressure relief, improved mobility, and weight tracking; a bariatric commode for when he is able to transfer; and a bariatric wheelchair to access his home. Mechanical assists for positioning are challenging for weights over 250 lbs., although ceiling-mounted lifts can support greater weights. Most scales have a maximum weight of 300 lbs. necessitating a specialized bariatric scale. A bariatric scale is useful for patients who can stand in order to track weight loss and manage diuresis in people with congestive heart failure. For people who need scale but cannot stand, an in-bed scale provides a method for following weights.

To obtain bariatric equipment through Medicare, durable medical equipment (DME) orders require a diagnosis, a weight over 250 lbs., and specific language addressing functional impact. Such language may include "Patient cannot ambulate 100 ft with use of cane, crutch, or walker due to morbid obesity (Dx E66.01; Z68.4x). Patient able to self-propel. Will benefit from wheelchair to complete ADLs within home." The two ICD-10 diagnoses identify morbid obesity (E66.01) and the body mass index over 40 (Z68.4x, with x varying by the BMI category).

Mr. X likely has sleep apnea and has been repeatedly hospitalized for hypercapnic respiratory failure. He was prescribed oxygen therapy at discharge but was not provided with a ventilation-support device, which he was to arrange "as an outpatient." While the hospitalist and pulmonary medicine consultant felt he needed chronic bi-level positive airway pressure (BiPAP) for adequate ventilation, Medicare guidelines require a sleep study before supplying BiPAP. Some respiratory suppliers can perform in-home sleep studies, which use nocturnal oximetry, and have a positive predictive value of 97% for identifying sleep apnea. Home sleep studies satisfy criteria to obtain a nocturnal ventilator assist device.

Management

Weight loss is a key element of Mr. X's treatment plan. Evidence on successful weight loss is limited in most populations. Dietary services in the home are similarly limited. Some mobility and exercise are important to maintain muscle mass. Morbidly obese individuals who are bedbound lose metabolically active muscle (sarcopenic obesity), thus reducing further their basal metabolic demand [1].

Bariatric surgery has been an effective intervention for morbid obesity, using one of two different techniques: gastric bypass and gastric sleeve. A recent systematic review found gastric bypass and gastric sleeve procedures more effective than gastric banding, with an average loss of 12–17 BMI points. Risks included a 17% complication and a 7% reoperation rate. Smaller studies focused on high-risk, older morbidly obese individuals also reported low mortality (<1%), with slightly higher complication rates (21%) [2, 3].

Even for the patient who desires definitive treatment and considers the 20% risk of complications worth the benefit, meeting criteria for bariatric surgery can be challenging for a homebound patient. Many insurers and bariatric surgery programs themselves require successful completion of 3–6 months of dietary nutrition classes. One potential solution is virtual learning, and facilitated virtual visits between home-based medical providers and center-based bariatricians are one potential intervention to traverse this gap, which some Medicare Advantage plans are exploring.

For patients who want to improve mobility without the risks of surgery, a physical therapy and occupational therapy evaluation can assist in teaching caregivers and patients how to meet their functional needs such as bed mobility, bathing, and proper skin care to manage risks of infection and breakdown, as well as developing a regular exercise program. Managing dietary intake is a challenge, as family and outside caregivers often purchase and prepare the meals. Family dynamics may make restrictive diets challenging. Simple, culturally sensitive food suggestions may be helpful, in conjunction with regular exercise.

Outcome

Mr. X obtained a bariatric bed and ceiling-mounted lift, which helped him increase his bed mobility, as well as his ability to sit up and work on improving his ability to transfer to a wheelchair. His nocturnal oximetry study confirmed multiple nocturnal desaturations, qualifying him for nocturnal ventilator assistance. He obtained an auto-adjusting BiPAP device, with wireless connection to his office-based pulmonologist.

The BiPAP device, however, had no oxygen adapter, requiring the patient to switch his oxygen supply to his BiPAP at night. He did not want bariatric surgery but with his increased mobility tried to go out to a local YMCA for aqua therapy, which was ultimately unsuccessful in promoting weight loss.

Clinical Pearls and Pitfalls

- Home-based medical care can provide dignified access to care and facilitate addressing specific obesity-related issues.
- Obesity leads to multiple medical complications, but immobility is a risk that can be mitigated with proper supportive equipment.
- In-home oximetry studies can be used to obtain nocturnal ventilator support, although insurance guidelines can make obtaining such devices challenging.
- DME contractors require specific language in a progress note to provide coverage for bariatric DME.

References

1. Cetin DC, Gaelle N. Obesity in the elderly: more complicated than you think. Cleve Clin J Med. 2014;81:51–61.
2. Chang SU, Stoll CRT, Song J, et al. The effectiveness and risks of bariatric surgery: an updated systematic review and meta-analysis 2003–2012. JAMA Surg. 2014;149:275–87.
3. Willkomm CM, Fisher TL, Barnes GS, et al. Surgical weight loss >65 years old: is it worth the risk? Surg Obes Relat Dis. 2010;6:491–6.

Chapter 19
Urinary Catheter Management at Home

**Rachel Kaplan, Karen Abrashkin,
and Konstantinos Deligiannidis**

Case Study

You make a home visit to Ms. Y, a 39-year-old woman with Chiari malformation type 1, spina bifida, type 2 diabetes, hypertension, and neurogenic bladder with chronic urinary retention, for complaints of abdominal discomfort. Ms. Y is homebound due to mild intellectual disability and wheelchair use for mobility. She lives in the basement of her parents' home and does not need assistance with her activities of daily living.

Ms. Y reports abdominal pain as soreness in the lower abdomen and rates her pain as 4 out of 10 on the pain scale. She denies fevers, chills, malaise, or flank pain. Until last year, she managed her urinary retention with a chronic indwelling urinary catheter, but she developed multiple complications, including frequent catheter-associated urinary tract infections (CAUTIs), necessitating a suprapubic catheter. Ms. Y uses a

R. Kaplan · K. Abrashkin · K. Deligiannidis (✉)
Northwell Health House Calls Program, New Hyde Park, NY, USA
e-mail: rkaplan3@northwell.edu; Kabrashkin@northwell.edu;
kdeligiann@northwell.edu

© Springer Nature Switzerland AG 2020
J. L. Colburn et al. (eds.), *Home-Based Medical Care for Older Adults*, https://doi.org/10.1007/978-3-030-23483-6_19

size 16-French urinary catheter and has experienced high levels of sediment production both with her indwelling urinary catheter as well as with the suprapubic catheter.

On examination, Ms. Y's vital signs are 146/86 mm Hg, heart rate 90 beats per minute, temperature 98.2 °F, and 16 respirations per minute. Her cardiopulmonary exam is normal. Her abdomen is sore to palpation in the suprapubic area without rebound tenderness or guarding; she has no costovertebral angle pain. She has no spasticity. Inspection of the suprapubic catheter reveals copious amounts of sediment encrusting the tubing. The urine output in the leg bag has significantly decreased over the past 24 hours. There is no erythema or skin breakdown surrounding the suprapubic site. Ms. Y states she feels anxious and she is adamant that she does not wish to go to the emergency department.

My Management

Which of the following is the next best step in management?

A. Prescribe ciprofloxacin for empiric treatment of CAUTI.
B. Send Ms. Y to the emergency department for revision surgery of the suprapubic site.
C. Exchange the suprapubic catheter in the home.
D. Irrigate the suprapubic catheter with normal saline.
E. Prescribe cephalexin daily for CAUTI prophylaxis.
F. Prescribe diazepam for anxiety related to catheter malfunction and bladder spasticity.

The correct answer is: C

Diagnosis and Assessment

Although Ms. Y has suprapubic soreness, she does not have fevers, chills, flank pain, or pyuria, which would be consistent with CAUTI. In patients with neurologic disease or spinal cord injury, malaise, autonomic hyperreflexia, or increased spasticity of the bladder can be signs of CAUTI, but she does not exhibit these symptoms [1]. The presence of sediment does not indicate an infection. Although a larger catheter (e.g., 18F) would decrease resistance and improve urinary flow [2], sending Ms. Y for revision surgery is not the best immediate step in management but could be considered in the future. If Ms. Y has not developed any outward signs of infection, and the supplies to change the catheter are not available, irrigating the catheter one or more times to ensure there is no obstruction is appropriate. If catheter irrigation is not successful, the suprapubic catheter should be exchanged, and recommend initiating weekly catheter irrigation to prevent future catheter clogging. If the output from the catheter has significantly decreased, as occurred with Ms. Y, then the suprapubic catheter will need to be changed. Antibiotic prophylaxis for CAUTI is not indicated at this time. Although diazepam may help with situational anxiety and spasticity, it is not appropriate first-line treatment and will not address the underlying condition.

Management

Urinary catheter care in the homebound individual is typically accomplished through a partnership between a skilled home health nurse, home-based medical care provider (sometimes with input from urologist), and with inclusion of the patient and caregiver in the care team. In most cases, home health nurses provide routine and urgent urinary catheter care; in some cases, home-based primary care providers may provide catheter changes on a routine or as-needed basis. Although suprapubic catheters are changed every 4–6 weeks [3], even up to a maximum of 12 weeks [4], some literature advocates for avoiding catheter changes if there are no problems with obstruction or infection [5].

The patient and the medical professionals managing the catheter must ensure that the stoma is clean and the catheter is irrigated (also called flushed) on a regular basis to avoid infection and/or obstruction. The catheter should be irrigated with 10 mL of normal saline at least once a week but also on an as-needed basis when sediment is seen in tubing or when output has decreased. Irrigating the catheter is accomplished by disconnecting the urinary catheter from the drainage bag, emptying the urine from the bladder using a sterile syringe, inserting a cleansing liquid (most commonly 10–60 cc normal saline) into the bladder via the side port of the catheter, and draining the saline [3].

Most often catheter care is performed by clinicians (registered nurses, primary care providers), but caregivers and patients can be trained to flush urinary catheters. Patients and caregivers should be alerted to signs of tube malfunction, including location of pain, tube dislodging, or clogging, in addition to signs of infection. Access to nursing and provider support is important in troubleshooting malfunctions telephonically or in person.

The presence of skin breakdown around the stoma is another concern. Caregivers must clean the stoma and protect the surrounding skin to prevent excoriation, maceration, irritation, and infection. Of note, physicians may not learn about the practical aspects of urinary catheter care in traditional medical training; for this reason it is particularly important to work with the entire care team in care of the homebound individual with an indwelling urinary catheter.

Outcome

Ms. Y's catheter was primarily managed by home health nursing with orders written by her home-based medical care provider. After building a rapport with the patient and developing a routine, Ms. Y's situational anxiety eased, and she allowed one specific home care RN to change her appliance monthly. The RN developed a routine approach with the patient to facilitate care. After arriving, the RN would slowly remove the soiled catheter, clean the stoma, assess the surrounding skin, and then reinsert the new catheter. The patient's parents were trained to flush the catheter with 10 mL normal saline at least once a week and change the bag routinely. Now comfortable with her catheter care, Ms. Y no longer experiences frequent complications.

Clinical Pearls and Pitfalls

- For patients with spinal cord injuries or neurologic disease, provide anticipatory guidance on lower urinary tract dysfunction and symptoms such as increased spasticity, sense of unease, or autonomic hyperreflexia [1].
- The presence of sediment in a urinary catheter does not mean that a patient has a urinary tract infection but may require more frequent flushing of a catheter to prevent obstruction.
- Troubleshooting urinary catheter malfunction telephonically or in person is an important skill for home-based medical providers.
- In the absence of urinary obstruction, or in a situation where a spare catheter is not available, irrigating the catheter one or more times to ensure there is no obstruction is appropriate.

References

1. Hooton TM, Bradley SF, Cardenas DD, et al. Diagnosis, prevention, and treatment of catheter-associated urinary tract infection in adults: 2009 international clinical practice guidelines from the Infectious Diseases Society of America. Clin Infect Dis. 2010;50(5):625–63.
2. Lee C, Gill BC, Vasavada SP, et al. Does size matter? Measured and modeled effects of suprapubic catheter size on urinary flow. Urology. 2017;102:266.e1–5.
3. MedlinePlus. Suprapubic catheter care. Online: https://medlineplus.gov/ency/patientinstructions/000145.htm. Accessed 3 Jan 2019.

4. Senese V, Hendricks MB, Morrison M, Harris J. Clinical practice guidelines: suprapubic catheter replacement. St. Louis: Society of Urologic Nurses and Associates; 2016. https://www.suna.org/sites/default/files/download/suprapubicCatheter.pdf. Accessed 11 Apr 2019.
5. Schaeffer AJ. Placement and management of urinary bladder catheters in adults. In: Richie JP, editor. UpToDate. 2017. https://www.uptodate.com/contents/placement-and-management-of-urinary-bladder-catheters-in-adults?search=suprapubic%20catheter§ionRank=1&usage_type=default&anchor=H10&source=machineLearning&selectedTitle=1~50&display_rank=1#H27. Accessed 3 Jan 2019.

Chapter 20
End-of-Life Care

Ina Li and Linsey O'Donnell

Case Study

You admit Ms. Z, a 92-year-old woman with a history of myocardial infarction, hypertension, seasonal allergies, and advanced Alzheimer's dementia, to your home-based medical care practice. Her medications include carvedilol, aspirin, clopidogrel, atorvastatin, and loratadine. She is oriented only to self and perseverates on the need to urinate. She is bedbound, incontinent of urine and feces, and is completely dependent on her daughter, who lives with her, for all basic and instrumental activities of daily living. She frequently and repetitively calls out "Help me!" during the day. Within the first few months of Ms. Z becoming your patient, she had multiple admissions to the emergency department and the hospital for changes in her mental status. Her daughter admits that when her mother begins to have any medical issues at home, in particular when she has increasing confusion, she becomes very anxious and calls 911.

I. Li (✉)
Clinical Director, Continuum of Care and Home Based Services, Christiana Care Health System, Wilmington, DE, USA
e-mail: ili@christianacare.org

L. O'Donnell
Clinical Lead, Community-based Supportive and Palliative Care Program, Christiana Care Health System, Wilmington, DE, USA

J. L. Colburn et al. (eds.), *Home-Based Medical Care for Older Adults*, https://doi.org/10.1007/978-3-030-23483-6_20

Multiple recent medical evaluations included head and abdominal CT scans, chest x-rays, an electroencephalogram (EEG), complete blood counts, comprehensive metabolic panels, and a thyroid stimulating hormone level. No significant abnormalities were noted on those evaluations. Her mental status changes have largely been attributed to urinary tract infection or constipation.

Despite treatment for suspected urinary tract infection with multiple courses of antibiotics, an adequate bowel regimen, and constant care by her daughter, Ms. Z's mental and functional status continues to decline. Her oral intake also starts to decline even with careful hand feeding by her daughter.

During your next house call, you review Ms. Z's recent history and situation with her daughter, who wants to do the best for her mother and have her lead as good of a life as possible. She also expresses frustration with the multiple emergency department and hospital visits and asks you what should be done to help Ms. Z.

My Management

Which of the following should you recommend?

A. Cystoscopy to determine etiology of recurrent urinary tract infection.
B. Add quetiapine to help with the patient's confusion and agitation.
C. Discuss Ms. Z's goals of care and prognosis with her daughter.
D. Tell the patient's daughter that the only option is referral to hospice.

Diagnosis and Assessment

The correct answer is C. It is essential to determine Ms. Z's prognosis. Utilizing a communications framework will help guide the goals of care discussion with her daughter, as you work together to develop an appropriate care plan.

Prescribing an antipsychotic medication is not the ideal initial step. Rather, the next step would be to have a goals of care discussion during which you can educate Ms. Z's daughter on common symptoms of dementia and non-pharmacologic options for management.

Further escalation to cystoscopy is not necessary. Please see Chap. 5 for a discussion of urinary tract infections.

Recommending hospice without having a goals of care discussion is unlikely to help the daughter understand her mother's condition and prognosis.

Management

Ms. Z's management starts with an assessment of prognosis. The Functional Assessment Staging Test (FAST) is validated in people with dementia and often used by hospice agencies for this purpose. Ms. Z is at a FAST Stage 7C, with the hallmarks of being unable to walk independently and with limited speech (see Table 20.1). At this stage, survival is often 6 months or less, and patients are hospice-appropriate [1].

Another simple prognostic tool is the "surprise question": "Would I be *surprised* if this patient *died* in the next 12 months?" For patients with advanced illnesses—such as dementia, end-stage renal disease, or heart failure—the sensitivity of an affirmative answer is approximately 75% [2]. Given Ms. Z's advanced dementia and her steady decline, most providers would not be surprised if Ms. Z died within the next 12 months. Both pieces of information inform a goals-of-care discussion with Ms. Z.'s daughter.

A goals-of-care discussion was held in the patient's home with Ms. Z and her daughter. Having this conversation can be very effective in the home setting. After determining Ms. Z.'s prognosis and reviewing her recent clinical course, the provider utilized the "Ask-Tell-Ask" communication approach [3] with Ms. Z.'s daughter to guide our discussion of goals of care.

TABLE 20.1 Functional Assessment Staging (FAST)

FAST Stage

1. No functional change

2. Subjective word difficulties

3. Decreased function in demanding work settings

4. Decreased ability to handle complex tasks such as finances

5. Requires assistance in choosing proper clothing

6. Moderately severe disease
   (a) Difficulty dressing properly
   (b) Requires assistance bathing
   (c) Inability to handle mechanics of toileting
   (d) Urinary incontinence
   (e) Fecal incontinence

7. Severe disease
   (a) Ability to speak limited to around six words
   (b) Intelligible vocabulary limited to a single word
   (c) Ambulatory ability lost
   (d) Ability to sit up lost
   (e) Ability to smile lost
   (f) Ability to hold head up lost

- The provider first *asked* what Ms. Z's daughter knew about her mother's condition. She told us "Mom is not able to do as much as before. The hospital is not making her better."
- The provider then used simple language to *tell* Ms. Z's daughter the medical information that needed to be conveyed stressing that her that her mother has advanced dementia and her medical status will continue to decline. The provider reassured her that it would be reasonable at this time to focus on quality of life rather than continuing hospitalizations and that that they would continue to be her doctors and visit her at home.
- The provider then *asked* her to summarize our recommendation to assess for understanding.

Ms. Z's daughter did not initially grasp that more hospitalizations would not lead to increased longevity or better quality of life for the patient. Ms. Z's daughter had many questions with each visit, and it was only after many hours of education and counseling that her daughter identified that both quality of life and being at home as much as possible were her primary priorities for her mother's goals of care. She understood and embraced the concept that medical treatments should only be performed if they would enhance her mother's quality of life, and our focus could now shift to providing Ms. Z maximal comfort in her own home. Medicare has advance care planning (ACP) billing codes to compensate medical providers for the extra time spent with the patient and family in reviewing goals of care [4].

Home-based medical care providers should be comfortable with implementing primary palliative care principles including symptom assessment, communication, and prognostication. For difficult cases, specialty-level palliative care consultation may be helpful if it is available in your community [5, 6].

Hospice, in contrast to palliative care, is a specific Medicare benefit that provides additional support focused toward comfort and quality of life in the last 6 months of life. Hospice can be administered in the home, or, if symptoms are severe, in an inpatient setting. Often support consists of nursing visits, personal aides a few times a week, social work, and chaplaincy. A patient cannot simultaneously receive Medicare skilled home health and hospice.

Given that Ms. Z. had a FAST score of 7C with a prognosis of 6 months or less, it was appropriate to approach her daughter about enrolling her into a hospice program. She told the providers that Ms. Z had instructed her in the past that she wanted to live at home as long as possible and "never wanted to live on machines." She agreed to home hospice.

The providers also worked with Ms. Z's daughter to complete a Physician's Orders for Life-Sustaining Treatment (POLST) form [7]. POLST is a medical order that details the specific medical treatments a patient would want during a medical emergency (such as resuscitation or hospital transfer). The title of a POLST form may differ between states, using other acronyms such as MOLST or POST. It can be completed with a surrogate and does not require the patient to have decision-making capacity to complete. Ms. Z's daughter is her designated health-care power of attorney, and she decided to choose do not resuscitate/do not intubate (DNR/DNI) and do not hospitalize status.

Outcome

Our home-based medical care providers continued to see Ms. Z. on a regular basis and serve as her primary medical team, with the hospice team seeing the patient on a weekly basis. Ms. Z.'s comfort was at the center of her care plan. Given that Ms. Z. was now enrolled in hospice, visits were billed using Medicare GV modifier for services related to her terminal diagnosis and GW for services not related to hospice diagnosis [8]. Carvedilol, aspirin, and clopidogrel were discontinued, as the survival benefit of these medications was negligible given Ms. Z's overall prognosis.

Hospice provided services that benefited both Ms. Z. and her daughter. Her daughter was comforted by the weekly nursing visits as Ms. Z.'s medical conditions were assessed and addressed in a timely fashion. The nurses continued to educate her on the course of advanced dementia so that she could proactively anticipate Ms. Z.'s needs and decline. For any urgent medical issues, Ms. Z's daughter called hospice, which often prompted an immediate home visit, assessment, and treatment of the issue. In addition, hospice provided home health aides to help with care and enabled her daughter to have some personal time to help ward off caregiver burnout. At one point, the hospice social worker arranged for Ms. Z. to receive respite care in an area nursing home so her daughter could take a vacation.

Ms. Z. declined slowly over the course of 2 years before dying peacefully at home in her sleep. Hospice provided bereavement services to support her daughter through this transition period.

Clinical Pearls and Pitfalls

- Utilize the FAST tool and the "surprise question" to help determine prognosis for patients with dementia.
- Use talking maps like "Ask-Tell-Ask" when communicating difficult news to a patient or family.
- Home-based medical care providers should be skilled in primary palliative care in the home setting. Referral to specialty-trained palliative medicine consultants is appropriate for refractory symptoms.
- Referrals to hospice care are appropriate when patients have a prognosis of 6 months or less and the goals of care center around quality of life and comfort.

References

1. Brown MA, Sampson EL, Jones L, Barron AM. Prognostic indicators of 6-month mortality in elderly people with advanced dementia: a systematic review. Palliat Med. 2013;27(5):389–400.
2. White N, Kupeli N, Vickerstaff V, Stone P. How accurate is the 'surprise question' at identifying patients at the end of life? A systematic review and meta-analysis. BMC Med. 2017;15(1):139.
3. Evans WG, Tulsky JA, Back AL, Arnold RM. Communication at times of transitions: how to help patients cope with loss and re-define hope. Cancer J. 2006;12(5):417–24.
4. CMS Medicare Learning Network Fact Sheet on Advance Care Planning. 2018. https://www.cms.gov/Outreach-and-Education/Medicare-Learning-Network-MLN/MLNProducts/Downloads/AdvanceCarePlanning.pdf. Accessed 11 Apr 2019.
5. Ritchie C, Leff B, Twaddle, M. My Favorite Slide: The Intersection of Home-Based Primary Care and Home-Based Palliative Care. 2017. https://catalyst.nejm.org/intersection-home-based-primary-care-palliative/. Accessed 11 Apr 2019.
6. Kavalieratos D, Corbelli J, Zhang D, et al. Association between palliative care and patient and caregiver outcomes: a systematic review and meta-analysis. JAMA. 2016;316(20):2104–14.
7. The National POLST Paradigm. http://polst.org/advance-care-planning/polst-and-advance-directives/. Accessed 11 Apr 2019.

8. CMS Medicare Learning Network Fact sheet on Hospice Related Services. 2014. https://www.cms.gov/Outreach-and-Education/Medicare-Learning-Network-MLN/MLNMattersArticles/Downloads/SE1321.pdf. Accessed 11 Apr 2019.

Additional Resources

Center to Advance Palliative Care (www.capc.org)
Fast Facts (www.mypcnow.org/fast-facts)

Index

© Springer Nature Switzerland AG 2020

139

J. L. Colburn et al. (eds.), *Home-Based Medical Care for Older
Adults*, https://doi.org/10.1007/978-3-030-23483-6

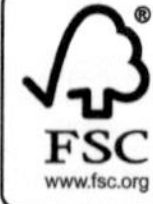